D1523944

Diversity in the Neuronal Machine

DIVERSITY IN THE NEURONAL MACHINE

Order and Variability in Interneuronal Microcircuits

Ivan Soltesz, Ph.D.
Department of Anatomy and Neurobiology
University of California, Irvine
Irvine, California

OXFORD
UNIVERSITY PRESS
2006

OXFORD

UNIVERSITY PRESS

Oxford University Press, Inc., publishes works that further
Oxford University's objective of excellence
in research, scholarship, and education.

Oxford New York
Auckland Cape Town Dar es Salaam Hong Kong Karachi
Kuala Lumpur Madrid Melbourne Mexico City Nairobi
New Delhi Shanghai Taipei Toronto

With offices in
Argentina Austria Brazil Chile Czech Republic France Greece
Guatemala Hungary Italy Japan Poland Portugal Singapore
South Korea Switzerland Thailand Turkey Ukraine Vietnam

Copyright © 2006 by Oxford University Press, Inc.

Published by Oxford University Press, Inc.
198 Madison Avenue, New York, New York 10016
www.oup.com

Oxford is a registered trademark of Oxford University Press

Library of Congress Cataloging-in-Publication Data
Soltesz, Ivan.
  Diversity in the neuronal machine : order and variability
  in interneuronal microcircuits Ivan Soltesz.
      p. ; cm.
  Includes bibliographical references and index.
  ISBN-13: 978-0-19-517701-5
  ISBN-0-19-517701-0
  1. Interneurons. 2. Neural networks (Neurobiology)
  [DNLM: 1. Interneurons—classification. 2. Hippocampus.
3. Interneurons—physiology. 4. Nerve Net—physiology. WL 102.5 S691d 2006] I. Title.
QP363.3.S535 2006
612.8'2—dc22   2005009389

9 8 7 6 5 4 3 2 1
Printed in the United States of America
on acid-free paper

To My Parents and Susie

Presumptuous man! Because your dim eyes
see only jumbled groupings there below,
you think that order and cooperation
do not exist in the workshop of life?
See for a moment how we spirits see,
And note what all their work achieves . . .

Lucifer, in *"The Tragedy of Man"* by I. Madach (1862)

Preface

It has been long recognized that neuronal networks in the mammalian brain consist of the numerically dominant, relatively homogenous, "principal" cells, and the less abundant, but much more diverse group of cells collectively referred to as interneurons. Since the pioneering studies by the great neuroanatomist Ramón y Cajal, a major strategy aimed at understanding cortical microcircuits has been to identify specific interneuronal subtypes, or "species," and try to assign distinct information processing functions to each of these groups. This research program, epitomized in the title of the famous book *The Cerebellum as a Neuronal Machine* (Eccles et al., 1967), has been phenomenally successful. Indeed, the basic idea that the different types of interneurons fit together to form a functioning nervous system, just as the cogs, nuts, and bolts make up a mechanical machine, continues to drive some of the greatest advances in research into cortical networks.

Within the past two decades, our understanding of interneuronal functions has dramatically improved. Specifically, it is now widely accepted that interneurons, which release the classical "inhibitory" neurotransmitter GABA, do far more than simple inhibition in neuronal networks. For example, interneurons generate various precisely controlled rhythms, the theta and gamma oscillations in the hippocampus that are associated with specific behaviors. Furthermore, partly due to drastically improved labeling techniques and the discovery of a long list of cell type–specific markers, our knowledge of the interneuronal constituents of various central nervous system areas has also increased. It is now widely accepted that each brain area is made of a certain number of interneuronal subtypes, each with a defining set of anatomical and physiological features. However, recent results also indicate that the emphasis on the highly specialized, distinct interneuronal cell classes alone cannot tell the whole story, because naturally occurring cellular variability between individual interneurons belonging to the same cell class can strongly modify the response properties and spontaneous oscillatory behaviors of neuronal networks. The major purpose of this book is to illustrate how discoveries concerning the functional relevance of the naturally existing cell-to-cell variability within defined interneuronal groups enrich the original ideas of the early pioneers on functional specialization. These new results show that diversity (the existence of many distinct interneuronal species) and variability (variance between individual cells within a given population of an interneuronal species) are two, mutually complementary, major characteristics of interneuronal networks, both of which are needed to fully understand the design principles underlying cortical circuits.

These ideas, as we shall see later, correspond well with the common experience of interneuronal researchers who encounter daily the Janus-faced nature of interneurons: the existence of highly specialized classes of cells with exquisite division of labor, and the simultaneous presence of cell-to-cell variability even within precisely defined interneuronal classes. The analogy with ecosystem and evolutionary theories can help to remind us of the general duality of biological order and variability: although understanding how ecosystems function requires the detailed studies of individual species and their interactions within a given ecosystem, however, adaptation and evolution could not occur without the existence of individual variability within the well-defined animal and plant species.

The ideas regarding interneuronal populations discussed in this book touch upon many important concepts in neuroscience, including the nature of hypothesized cortical processing units referred to as the canonical microcircuits, the necessity and limitations of the notion of neuronal "species," the duality of neuronal plasticity and homeostatic mechanisms, and the nature of the developmental processes and evolutionary constraints that may regulate the number and variance of interneuronal species. The book focuses primarily on a part of the cortex called the hippocampus, which is a brain area that is involved in learning and memory, spatial navigation, as well as in various neurological diseases. The hippocampus is also one of the most heavily researched brain areas, and its interneuronal populations are especially intensely studied. Therefore, the modern neuroscience of hippocampal interneurons gives us a uniquely rich source of detailed information that can be used to generate timely, comprehensive discussions on the role of order and variability in interneuronal microcircuits.

Currently, there is a tremendous and rapidly growing interest in interneuronal diversity. The landmark monograph published in a special edition of the journal *Hippocampus* by Freund and Buzsáki entitled "Hippocampal Interneurons" (commonly referred to as the "Bible" in most labs pursuing interneuronal research) in 1996 generated a wide readership and attention. The explosive growth of both our knowledge and the interest in this field since the Freund and Buzsáki review was highlighted by a series of review articles devoted to interneuronal diversity in 2003–2004 in the journal *Trends in Neurosciences*. As the first article in this series pointed out, "since 1995, the interneuron field has been growing more than three times as fast as the whole field of biomedical research, as judged by the number of interneuron-related papers appearing in MEDLINE, compared with the growth of MEDLINE itself" (Mott & Dingledine, 2003). It should be emphasized that the current book does not aim to cover all aspects of interneuronal anatomy and physiology. Instead, it focuses on a single theme, namely, on the nature of the dichotomy between the existence of specialized interneuronal classes and the natural variability within these distinct interneuronal populations.

The target audiences of this book are graduate students, postdoctoral fellows, and researchers interested in how neuronal networks function. Although the primary readership is likely to be the neuroscience community, the book is hopefully written in a scientifically rigorous yet easily readable style that should make it accessible to general biology undergraduates, as well as to computer engineers, computational modelers, and physicists interested in neuronal network theory. In addition, because the text contains several sections with relevance to alterations in interneuronal diversity in pathological states such as epilepsy, memory disturbances, and trauma, the book should be of interest to clinically oriented basic scientists working on mechanisms of neurological diseases as well.

Acknowledgments

No scientist works in isolation, and no monograph is really written by a single author. The latter is especially true for this book. Indeed, the idea for this book could not have been conceived without two decades of high-IQ (and often low-pH) inputs from many people. I would especially like to thank Tamás Freund and Peter Somogyi, who first drew my attention to the exquisite order that exists in interneuronal diversity. In-depth discussions with Peter in the past 5 years were particularly crucial for the crystallization and evolution of my early, rather fuzzy ideas regarding interneuronal variability into something more sharpened and substantial. As an added benefit of my studies with Tamás in Budapest, I had the good fortune to attend some of János Szentágothai's lectures on neuronal microcircuits at the Anatomy Institute in the 1980s, which were delivered in his characteristic, endlessly entertaining and deliriously inspiring style, in an effortless combination of German, French, English, and Hungarian (talk about order in diversity!).

I am indebted to all of those outstanding scientists that I worked with on various projects relating to the topic of this book, especially Ildiko Aradi, Viji Santhakumar, Csaba Földy, Jonas Dyhrfjeld-Johnsen, and Allyson Howard (who also provided generous and much appreciated assistance with the figures). Ildiko's novel ideas on variability left a particularly deep mark on my thinking about interneuronal species. Many thanks also to Edward G. Jones, who provided crucial insights and pointers regarding Cajal's research methods and historical aspects of interneuronal research. Interactions with many other neuroscientists over the years were also invaluable, and I would like to specifically thank Richard Miles, Roger Traub, Gyuri Buzsáki, Alex Thomson, Attila Gulyás, Mircea Steriade, Zoltan Nusser, Chris McBain, Gabor Tamas, Martin Deschênes, Istvan Mody, Peter Jonas, Katalin Toth, Vincenzo

Crunelli, Laszlo Acsády, Norbert Hájos, and the late Eberhard Buhl for their contributions to shaping my thinking about this problem. The core ideas of this book have been field- and sometimes battle-tested in conversations with many other scientists, including Charles Stevens, Larry Abbott, Thomas Carew, Terry Sejnowski, Jean-Marc Fellous, Paul Tiesinga, X.-J. Wang, Eve Marder, John Rubenstein, Ole Paulsen, Christophe Bernard, Kai Kaila, Miles Whittington, Fiona LeBeau, and Sacha Nelson. Discussions with Georg Striedter, Hans Hofmann, and Eörs Szathmáry were important for my thinking regarding interneuronal heterogeneity and evolution. Thanks to Miriam Meisler for pointing out to me several key publications on somatic mutation rates, to Matthew Turner for detailed advice on statistics, and to Péter Érdi and László Záborszky for their advice regarding Szentágothai's and Rényi's studies.

I want to also thank those past and present members of my laboratory whom I have not yet mentioned, especially Anna Ratzliff, Steven Ross, Julio Echegoyen, Kang Chen, Axel Neu, Robert Morgan, and Rose Zhu, who not only contributed to many of the research projects that led to this book but also did not complain when I sequestered myself someplace to selfishly work on this monograph instead of being in the lab with them—you guys were great!

I would also like to express my love and gratitude to my wife Susie Hsieh, for her constant support and encouragement, and for braving the myriad forms of bloodthirsty bugs (not to mention the equally diverse effects of certain prophylactic medications against tropical diseases) in various rain forests of the world as she accompanied me in my quest to understand the parallels between ecosystem theory, island biogeography, and neuronal microcircuits.

Finally, I want to thank the National Institute for Neurological Diseases and Stroke (NINDS; grant numbers NS38580 and NS35915) for the financial support that made it possible for our laboratory at UC Irvine to pursue our research interests on interneuronal functions in normal and pathological states.

Contents

Contents   xvii

Diversity in the Neuronal Machine

1

Introduction

> *... pyramidal cells, like the plant in a garden—as it were, a series of*
> *hyacinths—are lined up in hedges which describe graceful curves.*
> S. Ramón y Cajal (1989)

A Walk in the Neuronal Forest

Before we begin our discussions about order and variability in
interneuronal microcircuits in earnest, let's stretch our legs a bit by
taking a brief walk in a neuronal forest. First, let's gather the essential gear for our hike. Because we do not have a wireless neuronal
GPS device, we just have to look up the bregma-centric coordinates
for Ammon's Horn in the hippocampus the old-fashioned way, by
thumbing through the coffee-stained brain atlas from the lab. Let's
make sure that we have a flashlight ("torch," for those who speak
English) to peer into dark spaces, and a rope with a harness to
climb trees. Let's grab our precious copy of the interneuronal
researchers' "Bible" (Freund & Buzsáki, 1996) to help us identify the
rarer interneuronal species that we encounter on our journey, and
we are ready to enter the magical land (Fig. 1.1).

As we look around, we first notice the orderly, long, black rows of
the massive trunks of the pyramidal trees. Immediately, it is evident
that these creatures are by far the most abundant, numerically dominant species in the forest. We crank our necks to look up and mar-
vel at the majestic main vertical branches of these fabulous trees,
rising high toward the sky. Soon, as our eyes adjust to the twilight
in the deep forest, we realize that the apical trunk high above suddenly gives rise to thinner distal branches that form a wide canopy,
just like the giant trees in the rain forests of Costa Rica. As we continue our leisurely stroll, we start to notice some of the less abundant

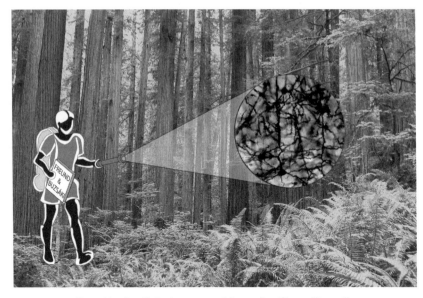

Figure 1.1   **A walk in the neuronal forest** (by Allyson Howard).

inhabitants. In fact, after a while, we realize that there are many different species everywhere around us, hidden among the pyramidal trees. Long, convoluted, basket-like tentacles of a curious species crawl around the base of the pyramidal trees and climb up on lower portions of the apical trunk. As we direct our attention to what is below our feet, in places where the earth has been washed away we notice an oddball creature hiding among the basal dendrites of the giant pyramids. We shine our flashlight on it and follow its tentacles and realize that it belongs to a ground-dwelling species whose main characteristic feature is a long, virtually vertical branch that disappear in the distant canopy. We take a deep breath, give a quick prayer to the patron saint whom Cajal considered his own, Santiago (St. James) the apostle (Cajal, 1989), and hoist ourselves up into the canopy with the rope. Once we reach the distal branches, we notice that the canopy has its own specialized inhabitants, including some whose processes never leave the high altitudes. As we continue our exploration, depending on our luck and perseverance, we may encounter several more, perhaps even the rarest of the interneuronal species, each with its own, apparently well-defined niche.

Once we reach the end of our journey in this enchanted land, it is impossible not to be amazed by the extraordinary diversity of life in the neuronal forest. We leave the forest with a sense that this varied landscape holds many secrets. How do we determine the position, connectivity, abundance, and role of each individual component of this extraordinary, miniature ecosystem? How do we define interneuronal "species" in the first place? Exactly how many species make up this forest? How variable are the individuals that belong to a single species? How do the various species interact? How is a complex system, like the one we have just explored, put together from its individual constituents during its development, and how does it evolve across thousands and thousands of generations? How does the neuronal forest respond to perturbations such as the loss of rare species? I hope that these questions do not make you think of a "pleasant walk spoiled" (to use Mark Twain's words originally intended for golf), and you find these questions just as exciting as I have found them to be ever since I first peered through a microscope and got lost, mostly on purpose, in various parts of the neuronal forest. So let's begin to explore the extraordinary diversity of the enchanted world of interneurons.

Historical Roots: Nuts and Bolts of a Neuronal Machine

It was the Czech Jan Purkinje who, while working in Breslau (the present-day Wroclaw in Poland) in the 1820s, identified the first nerve cell type in the nervous system, the Purkinje cells of the cerebellum (note that the term "neuron" was not introduced until much later, in 1891 by Wilhelm von Waldeyer) (Shepherd, 1991). Purkinje was also the first to represent brain areas as being composed of distinct populations of nerve cells located in specific layers (Shepherd, 1991). Figure 1.2 shows one of the first published views of the cellular composition of a brain region, the cerebellum, from 1838, where Purkinje clearly distinguished the granule cells and the Purkinje cell populations. Because we will primarily focus on cortical microcircuits in this book, it should be mentioned that it was Albrecht von Kölliker in 1849 who first detected differences in the morphology of unstained neurons dissociated from the fixed human cerebral cortex, but it was Berlin in 1858 who, as explained by DeFelipe and Jones (1988), "first stained sections of the cortex with carmine and was able to discern not only the arrangement of its cells into layers but also the presence of three types of cells that he called

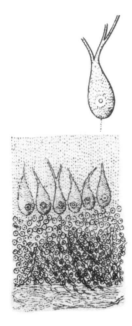

Figure I.2   **The first identified nerve cell in the nervous system**: the large corpuscles of the cerebellum, which became known as Purkinje cells after their discoverer. This was also the first published view of the cellular composition of the histological layers within a brain region. From below: fibers, granules, large corpuscles (Purkinje cells), molecular layer. Original in Purkyně (Purkinjé) Society (1937), *In Memoriam: Joh. Ev. Purkyne 1787–1937*; Prague: Purkyne Society. Reprinted, with permission, from Shepherd (1991).

pyramidal, fusiform or spindlelike, and grains or granules." It is noteworthy that these terms are used even today.

It was in 1873 that Camillo Golgi, Head Physician of the Hospice for Incurables in the small Italian town of Abbiategrasso, near Pavia, published his first results obtained with his "black reaction" staining technique in a paper in the Italian Medical Gazette entitled "On the structure of the gray matter of the brain." It was in this paper that Golgi, using his revolutionary silver-based staining method that allowed the visualization of fine axonal side branches, first distinguished type I cells, those with long axis cylinders (projection neurons), and type II cells, those with short axis cylinders (short-axon cells). The latter neurons include those cells that we now call GABAergic interneurons. What Golgi actually argued is that not every axon (using today's terminology originally introduced by Kölliker) joined the white matter, because some neurons had axons that ended within the particular brain locality where the cell bodies resided: "I can from now on refute the generally held opinion that it [the axon] always goes on to constitute the cylinder axis of the medullary nerve fibers; that is, at least, not the general rule." Later on, Golgi talks about the two types of "gangliar" cells in even more precise terms (Golgi, 1873):

In relation to the different mode of behavior of the nervous prolongation, in the gray substance of the nervous centers, two types of gangliar cells can be distinguished, viz:

    a. Gangliar cels whose nervous prolongation, though it gives off some lateral threads, maintains its proper individuality, and passes on to place itself in direct relation with the nervous fibres [cells of long axons].

    b. Gangliar cells whose nervous prolongation, subdividing complexly, loses its proper individuality and takes part in tot in the formation of a diffuse nervous network. These cells, therefore, would have only indirect relations with the nervous fibres [cells of short axon].

As the previous passage illustrates, Golgi believed that the local axons of the type II neurons all join together into a diffuse reticular network through anastomoses. Albeit not widely known, it could be a source of great pride to all interneuron researchers that Santiago Ramón y Cajal first argued against the reticular network theory in favor of the neuron doctrine using the example of the pattern of innervation by basket cell axons. The following passage is also the first detailed description of a bona fide interneuron, Cajal's "stellate cells," now known as the basket cells of the cerebellum (Cajal, 1888a; Shepherd, 1991):

... the special character of these cells is the unique arrangement of their nervous filament [axon]. This arises from the cell body ... runs for a considerable distance through the molecular layer, giving off numerous branches, some ascending and other descending .... The descending branches always arise at a certain vertical angle from the trajectory of the nervous prolongations; descending, they grow visibly thicker, ramify at acute angles, and terminate in fringes [tufts] of short and varicose fibers [baskets] which envelope completely the bodies of the Purkinje cells. Due to their abundance and thickness, these fringes form a virtual layer in the transition zone between the molecular layer and granular layers. The fibers that form them do not anastomose among themselves and, apparently, end freely ....

What's more (to inflate the pride of interneuronal researchers some more), it was also the example of the "fringes" (basket cell perisomatic axonal arrangements) that led Cajal to make the first step toward the principle of dynamic polarization; that is, that axons send nervous activity, and dendrites and somata receive them (Cajal, 1888b; from Shepherd, 1991; modified from Clarke and O'Malley, 1968):

> The contacts between [Purkinje cells] and the [descending fringes (i.e. basket endings)] are ... so numerous that it is possible to say that each of the Purkinje cells lies on a cushion of ramifications of the cylinder [axons]. Now then, could not these very extensive and intimate connections be the means which nature provides to allow the nerve current to pass from one cell to the other; for example, from the stellate [basket] cells that have hitherto been considered sensory, to those of Purkinje which have been supposed to be motor?

In addition to basket cells, Cajal recognized and distinguished a number of (what we now call) interneuronal cell types in cortical structures, including the neurogliaform cells, the double bouquet cells (for a photograph of such a cell from Cajal's own preparation, see Fig. 1.3), cells with ascending axons (partly corresponding to Martinotti cells), and a less well-defined group of cells with short axons (DeFelipe & Jones, 1988). Cajal was certainly not without illustrious scientific predecessors, such as the aforementioned Purkinje, Golgi, and Kölliker, as well as Otto Dieters, Wilhelm His, August Forel, Paul Ehrlich, Fridtjof Nansen, Michael von Lenhossék, and Gustav Retzius (for superb and highly entertaining historical accounts of these neuroscientists, see Clarke & Jacyna, 1987; DeFelipe & Jones, 1988; and Shepherd, 1991). Many of these scientists contributed hugely to the development of the neuron doctrine with a long series of brilliant technical advances and conceptual insights. However, it was undoubtedly Cajal himself who created a lasting scientific revolution that gave birth to a whole new field of neuroscience, known today as functional neuroanatomy. The long-term goal of Cajal's approach was to arrive at mechanistic explanations of brain functions, or, as he himself referred to it, lay the foundations of a "rational psychology" (Cajal, 1989; Nicoll, 1994). With his exquisite drawings of the cellular constituents of the nervous system (Cajal, 1909, 1911), Cajal demonstrated in hitherto unimagined and unparalleled details that each area of the nervous system contains specialized neuronal networks consisting of precisely defined, diverse cell types (a type of diversity that we will later refer to as alpha diversity), and that these cell types differ from each other

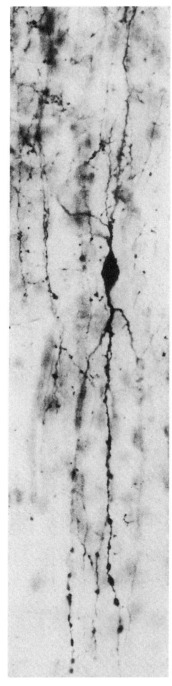

Figure 1.3 **Photomicrograph from one of Cajal's preparations**, showing a bitufted ("double bouquet") cell in layer III of the visual cortex of a 15-day-old human brain. ×430. Reprinted, with permission, from DeFelipe and Jones (1988).

according to position, connectivity, and, presumably, function. It was also Cajal who, building on Purkinje's and others' earlier work, demonstrated in the most detailed form that different brain areas, which serve different sensory, motor, or other functions, are composed of distinct cellular constituents, thus highlighting the importance of a type of neuronal diversity that we will refer to as beta diversity.

From the perspective of the main topics of this book, what Cajal's work implied, above all, was that the functions and behavior of nervous systems can be understood, perhaps all they way to psychology, once the structural and functional properties of its components are described and their connections are painstakingly determined, just like a mechanical device can be understood by describing its individual components and the rules by which these parts fit together. Or, as Cajal himself phrased it (Cajal, 1899; DeFelipe & Jones, 1988): "it is seen that the true understanding of cerebral activity will not be achieved until organ physiology has been transformed into histophysiology, changing the study of organic resultants into [that of] the elemental components."

This basic idea was implemented in the subsequent decades by a number of illustrious masters of functional neuroanatomy, such as Lorente de Nó during the 1920s and 1930s (for excellent historical assessments of the lasting impact of Cajal's observations, see DeFelipe & Jones, 1988; Shepherd, 1991; Jones, 1999). Increasingly, starting in the 1950s, neuroscientists took advantage of possibilities presented by electron microscopy–aided microanatomy that allowed the first resolution of the synaptic cleft (e.g., Palade & Palay, 1954), which put an end to all rearguard partisan arguments against the neuron doctrine (note that Cajal felt it necessary to publish in 1933, one year before his death, a renewed defense of his neuron doctrine in "Neuronismo o reticularismo?"; Shepherd, 1991). It was also the electron microscope that allowed the discovery and differentiation of asymmetric and symmetric synapses (Gray, 1961), which, in today's functional terms, largely corresponded to glutamatergic excitatory and GABAergic inhibitory synapses, respectively. In addition to the electron microscope, the second technical innovation that took hold around the 1950s was single-cell intracellular electrophysiology (in anesthetized preparations in vivo), resulting in the discovery of inhibitory postsynaptic potentials (IPSPs) following stimulation of interneurons (Brock et al., 1952; Coombs et al., 1955). It is interesting to note that Cajal himself never invoked "inhibition" in his discussions about neuronal networks (Shepherd, 1991), even though inhibitory nerve action was known by that time (e.g., inhibition of the heart by the vagus nerve and the inhibition of spinal reflexes by higher centers) (Jacobson, 1993).

As already mentioned earlier in the preface, an important, comprehensive functional neuroanatomy-based synthesis appeared during the 1960s with the rather explicit title *The Cerebellum as a Neuronal Machine* (Eccles et al., 1967). This book, based on a series of results obtained using an imaginative combination of electron microscopical and electrophysiological techniques, attested to the continued vitality of Cajal's research paradigm. The three authors, John Eccles, Masao Ito, and János Szentágothai, possessed different technical expertise, but they closely shared a common vision inspired by Cajal's functional neuroanatomical thinking. The authors all strived to understand cerebellar functions through a detailed description of the microscale connectivity pattern and response properties (as they put it in the book) "arising from all manner of inputs" of each individual cell types of the cerebellar cortex. The process of assembling of the neuronal machine from the individual components was described by Szentágothai in his Ferrier lecture (Szentágothai, 1978) this way:

> The basic mental strategy of assembling neuron networks from virtually completely stained but isolated individual cells, was that of looking for the "best spatial fitting" between terminal axon arborizations and potential postsynaptic sites, such as cell bodies, major dendrites and characteristic points of their arborizations, dendritic spines, etc.

It is interesting to note that, in the vision of Eccles and his colleagues, their investigations were primarily aimed at identifying the structural and functional properties of the individual components, and they proposed that it would be with the help of "theorists" that the computing machine would be eventually put together and fully explained. They closed their "Neuronal Machine" book with these inspiring words that ring true even today:

> It has been ... the guiding principle of the whole book that the cerebellum is a part of the brain with a design of neuronal connexions especially adapted for its function in the rapid and effective computation of information fed into it. In attempting to gain insight into the

way in which its neuronal structure can function as a computing machine it is essential to be guided by the insights that can be achieved by communication theorists and cyberneticists who have devoted themselves to a detailed study of cerebellar structure and function.

Functional neuroanatomy-based study programs were also successfully applied to microcircuits in various brain areas. Figure 1.4 illustrates one of Szentágothai's drawings of the cellular equivalents of the nuts and bolts for a single unit in the machinery of the cerebral cortex. There are two major concepts conveyed by Szentágothai's figure. First, the drawing suggests that the essence of the cortical microcircuit can be understood by determining the precise input–output connectivity and physiology (i.e., "function") of the individual cell types, such as the basket cells (BCs), axo-axonic cells (AACs), and the double bouquet cells (CDBs). For example, axo-axonic cells and basket cells are shown innervating specifically and exclusively the axon initial segments and somata of pyramidal cells, respectively, whereas the double bouquet cell is depicted as synapsing on the dendritic regions of postsynaptic cells. This almost crystal-like anatomical arrangement has implicit, direct functional relevance. For example, axo-axonic cells are in a prime position to control the generation of action potentials, whereas the double bouquet cells, by virtue of their preference for dendritic spines, are more likely to be able to gate individual, specific excitatory inputs. In addition to illustrating the cellular constituents of a neuronal machine, the drawing also depicts the idea of a cortical network unit or module, suggesting that the cortex consists of a more or less monotonous multiplication of this basic organizational entity. As we shall see throughout this book, these two major concepts in various, sometimes evident, other times more implicit forms, still provide some of the key intellectual underpinnings of cortical microcircuit theory. It is also interesting to point out that, based on comparative neuroanatomical observations in various species across the phylogenetic spectrum, it was widely believed that evolution built more complex machines from more diverse parts. Cajal thought that "the functional superiority of the human brain is intimately bound up with the prodigious abundance and unusual wealth of forms of the so-called neurons with short axons . . . ." (Cajal, 1989; DeFelipe & Jones, 1988). Because this latter fascinating issue is not entirely settled even today,

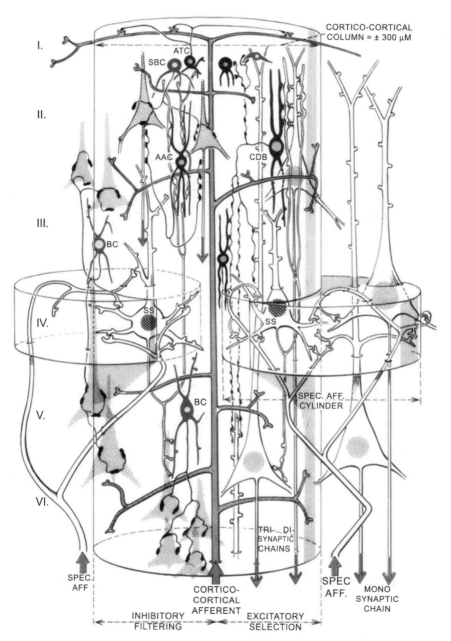

Figure 1.4 **Neuronal circuits of a representative corticortical column.** Cells drawn solid black or gray are cells that were known or assumed to be inhibitory in the early 1980s. SBC, small basket cell; AAC, axo-axonic (chandelier) cell; BC, basket cell; ATC, axonal tuft cell; CDB, double bouquet cell. Pyramidal cells and the spiny stellate cells (SS) are drawn in outline. Reprinted, with permission, from Szentágothai (1983).

13

we will discuss some of the evolutionary and circuit design–related implications of interneuronal diversity later in the book.

Great Victories of Cajal's "Rational Psychology" Paradigm

The enduring, fundamental veracity and power of Cajal's approach and insights were taken to even more impressive heights by the series of discoveries and breakthroughs that took place in the last two decades of the past century. The list of major victories of functional neuroanatomy is impressive, even if one concentrates only on those that specifically concerned neocortical and hippocampal interneurons. At the most fundamental level, the number of distinct interneuronal classes recognized and commonly accepted has dramatically increased, mostly because new, biocytin-based single-cell labeling techniques allowed the resolution of axonal and dendritic trees of interneurons (Fig. 1.5A) in a much richer detail than previously possible, leading to the better description of known cell classes and the discovery of new subtypes.

In the hippocampus, where the inputs are organized in an especially clearly delineated, layer-specific manner, the functional relevance of the dendritic and axonal patterns of interneuronal subtypes is especially easy to appreciate. In the case of the CA1 region, there are five major glutamatergic inputs that arrive in different layers or combination of layers. These include the numerically dominant input from the ipsi- and contralateral CA3 pyramidal cells to the stratum radiatum and oriens, the entorhinal input to the lacunosum-moleculare and oriens, the thalamic input to the lacunosum-moleculare, and the input from the CA1 pyramidal cells themselves and from the amygdala to the oriens. Thus, the distal dendritic lacunosum-moleculare layer (Fig. 1.5) is the major (but not exclusive) recipient of the entorhinal cortical (and thalamic) inputs. Inputs from the pyramidal cells located in the CA3 region form the Schaffer collateral pathway that resides in the CA1 stratum radiatum, where the more proximal dendritic branches of CA1 pyramidal cells are located. The axons from the CA1 pyramidal cells themselves exit the pyramidal cell layer and give off collaterals in the stratum oriens (Fig. 1.5A), where the basal dendrites of the CA1 pyramidal cells reside. In addition to innervating CA1 pyramidal cells, the major excitatory pathways also make synapses on the various types of CA1 interneurons. However, unlike the CA1 pyramidal cells whose dendrites span all layers, interneuronal types differ from each other with respect to the layers that their dendrites are located at, and, consequently, in the types of excitatory inputs they can sample. The layer-specific location of interneuronal dendrites is illustrated in Fig. 1.5B (note that a recent, more complete, although certainly not ultimate, listing of the known interneuronal species of CA1 will be discussed later; our point here in the introduction is to give a general idea of the major dendritic and axonal patterns and major cell-specific labels for the CA1 interneurons). Some interneurons have dendrites that reside in the stratum lacunosum-moleculare, where they sample the entorhinal activity, but these cells do not receive CA3 or CA1 pyramidal cell inputs. Others, such as the oriens–lacunosum-moleculare (OLM) cell shown in Fig. 1.5A, possess dendrites that are restricted to the stratum oriens. Such anatomical segregation of dendrites, therefore, determines the primary input of each of the specific types of interneuron in the network. In simple functional terms, the position of the dendrites determines whether some cells, like the interneurons residing in the lacunosum-moleculare layer, are activated by excitatory activity that arrive to the CA1 pyramidal cells from another brain area (e.g., the entorhinal cortex) in a "feed-forward" manner, or, like the OLM cells, are also activated in a feedback manner (i.e., following the discharge of the CA1 pyramidal cells themselves).

Similar to the layer-specific segregation of dendritic trees, different interneuronal subtypes innervate distinct parts of pyramidal cells. The axonal target-specificity is illustrated in the layer-specificity of the various interneuronal subtypes depicted in Fig. 1.5. Improvements in single cell visualization techniques especially enhanced our appreciation of the axonal output specificity, leading not only to a higher-resolution description of previously described cell types (e.g., basket cells, see Fig. 1.5A) but also to the discovery of a number of new interneuronal subtypes. For example, the bistratified cells (Buhl et al., 1994a) innervate the basal and apical dendritic regions of CA1 pyramidal cells, but their axons avoid the somatic cell layer (Fig. 1.5A), presenting a complementary innervation pattern to basket and axo-axonic cells. The long axons of OLM cells (Fig. 1.5A), streaming from the cell body located in the stratum oriens to the terminal arborization site in the lacunosum-moleculare, have also been better understood as a result of improved single cell visualization methods.

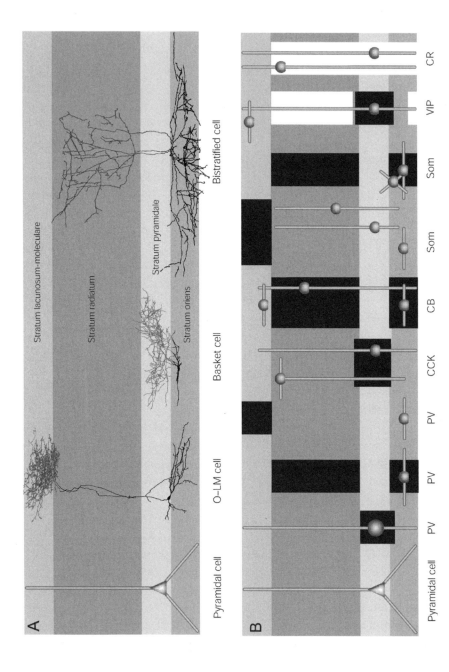

16

Figure 1.5 **Major interneuronal subtypes in the CA1 region of the hippocampus.** (A) Camera lucida reconstructions of three stratum oriens-alveus interneurons showing the domain-specific innervation of pyramidal cells by their axons. A stratum oriens–lacunosum-moleculare cell (OLM cell; for the original drawing of this cell with exact, nonstylized layer-specificity, see Maccaferri et al., 2000) projects its axon to pyramidal cell distal dendrites of the stratum lacunosum-moleculare. A basket cell soma, located within stratum oriens, projects its axon to the pyramidal neuron soma and the proximal dendrites. A bistratified cell sends its axon to both basal and apical dendrites in stratum oriens and radiatum. Far left, cartoon of a pyramidal cell showing the approximate location of the basal and apical dendrites and the cell body (original version of this figure appeared in Maccaferri et al., 2000). (B) The laminar distribution of dendritic and axonal arbors of different types of interneurons containing calcium-binding proteins and neuropeptides in the hippocampus. Circles mark the general soma location of each interneuron type. The lines emanating from them indicate the predominant orientation and laminar distribution of the dendritic tree. Black boxes represent the laminae where the axon of each interneuron type typically extends its arbor. White, vertically oriented boxes indicate that other interneurons, rather than principal cells, are the primary targets. The transverse extent of the dendrites or axon is not indicated. CB, calbindin; CCK, cholecystokinin; CR, calretinin; PV, parvalbumin; Som, somatostatin; VIP, vasoactive intestinal peptide. The original version of this figure appeared in Freund and Buzsáki (1996). Adapted, with permission, from McBain and Fisahn (2001).

In addition to improved resolution of the axonal and dendritic patterns, the combination of single cell visualization methods with a large number of excellent, cell-specific immunocytochemical markers also resulted in the fundamentally important recognition that there is frequent correlation between the axonal and dendritic characteristics on the one hand and the immunocytochemical identity on the other (Fig. 1.5B). Although the precise functional relevance of some of these markers is not always understood in detail, there are many examples where a receptor protein with a specific function, or a particular ion channel, have been shown to be expressed only in a subset of cells. As a result of these combined anatomical, physiological, and functional explorations, the number of anatomical interneuronal subtypes increased further. For example, instead of a single group of hippocampal basket cells, we now talk about parvalbumin- or cholecystokinin (CCK-) positive basket cells (Fig. 1.5B), as these two subclasses show a number of strictly segregated anatomical, physiological, and pharmacological properties (to be discussed later in detail in chapter 3).

The recognition of such functionally meaningful interneuronal categories, not just in the CA1 and the broader hippocampal formation, but also in many other cortical and subcortial areas, constitutes a living, constantly evolving memorial for Cajal's heritage. The high specificity of the axonal and dendritic patterns of distinct interneuron subtypes also resulted in the insight that there is likely to be a precisely defined, highly controlled, functionally important division of labor among the various interneurons (Han et al, 1993; Halasy et al., 1996), in the sense that each of the various microcircuit functions (e.g., feedback inhibition of distal dendrites, the inhibitory control of action potential initiation, etc.) is provided by a specialized, dedicated interneuronal subtype. In addition, modern functional neuroanatomy, working toward the ultimate goal of a "rational psychology," not only offered an ever-expanding list of interneuronal species, but it also proved itself able to move beyond its traditional boundaries by directly testing its predictive power.

A listing of some of the major discoveries concerning interneuronal microcircuits within the hippocampus and neocortex is presented below. Evidently, such a list is bound to be incomplete and somewhat subjective. Nevertheless, the list below aptly illustrates the tremendous advances that have been made toward understanding the neuronal machine.

1. Discovery of the most specialized type of interneuron known to date, the chandelier cells (Szentágothai & Arbib, 1974; Jones, 1975; for a recent review, see Howard et al., 2005). It is interesting that Cajal never described this cell type, perhaps because the axonal tree, the most characteristic feature of these cells, was not fully developed in the fetal and neonatal material that Cajal mostly studied (DeFelipe & Jones, 1988). These cells were so named by Szentágothai because the cartridges (vertical rows of axonal terminals) resemble candles on a chandelier. Subsequently, chandelier cells were shown to make symmetric synapses selectively on axon initial segments of pyramidal and granule cells in the neocortex and hippocampus (Somogyi, 1977; Somogyi et al., 1982; Peters et al., 1982), which led to the alternative term "axo-axonic cells" for chandelier cells. The specificity of these cells for the initial segment is typically, albeit not invariably, absolute.

2. Discovery that interneurons express certain neuropeptides (e.g., CCK and somatostatin; Somogyi et al., 1984), calcium-binding proteins (e.g., parvalbumin; Celio, 1986), receptors for neurotransmitters and neuromodulators (e.g., muscarinic type 2 receptors; Hajos et al., 1998; cannabinoid type 1 receptors; Katona et al., 1999b) cytoskeletal elements (e.g., neurofilament heavy; Ratzliff & Soltesz, 2000, 2001), and certain ion channels (e.g., P/Q-type Ca^{2+}-channels; Wilson et al., 2001) in a highly subtype-specific-manner.

3. Discovery that the GABAergic septo-hippocampal pathway exclusively innervates hippocampal GABAergic interneurons (Freund & Antal, 1988). The specificity of this GABA to GABA, long-distance connection comprises a key element of the disinhibitory mechanisms underlying the generation of the theta oscillations (Buzsáki et al., 1983; Soltesz & Deschênes, 1993; Toth et al., 1997b). The discovery of the target specificity of the septo-hippocampal pathway also led to research that resulted in the description of the high specificity of other input pathways; for example, the serotonergic input to hippocampal interneurons (Freund et al., 1990).

4. Discovery of interneurons that innervate specifically and exclusively other interneurons (Acsády et al., 1996b; Gulyás et al., 1996) (Fig. 1.6). This anatomical result indicated that

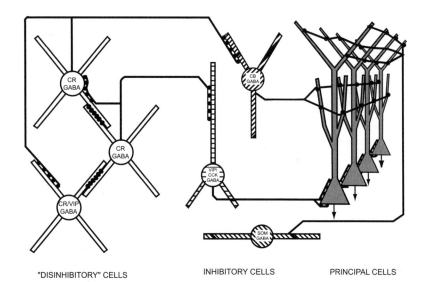

"DISINHIBITORY" CELLS INHIBITORY CELLS PRINCIPAL CELLS

Figure I.6 **Hippocampal microcircuits consist of three major components**: (1) the principal cells (gray cells) account for the majority of cortical cells and form long-range as well as local, excitatory connections; (2) diverse groups of inhibitory cells (hatchings), which control the activity of principal cells by exerting inhibition on different somato-dendritic domains; and (3) "disinhibitory" neurons (open cells). The calretinin-immunoreactive "disinhibitory" neurons are massively interconnected by dendro-dendritic (parallel bars on their dendrites) and axo-dendritic contacts with each other. As a result of mutual synaptic interconnection and dendritic coupling, the activity of these neurons is likely to become rhythmic and synchronized. This oscillation is then conveyed to large populations of pyramidal cells via different inhibitory cell populations. Both dendritic (CB-immunoreactive cells) and perisomatic (VIP/CCK-immunoreactive cells) inhibition of principal cells may be synchronized in this manner. It is important to note here that, for the sake of clarity, several components of the hippocampal inhibitory circuitry have been ignored to obtain this diagram. Other subsets of inhibitory cells (e.g., conventional basket cells) are also known to provide input to interneurons, although their major targets remain pyramidal cells. CR, calretinin; CB, calbindin D28k. Reprinted, with permission, from Gulyás et al. (1996).

these interneurons are likely to be in a prime position to control the activity of populations of other interneurons ("conductor cells"). Subsequently, other examples of interneuron-specific interneuron species have also been found (Gulyás et al., 2003).

5. Discovery that gap junctional, electrical contacts preferentially exist between interneurons belonging to the same subtype (Gibson et al., 1999; Galarreta & Hestrin, 1999, 2001; Beierlein et al., 2000; Tamas et al., 2000; Szabadics

et al., 2001). The existence of gap junctional coupling between specific interneuronal species is a great example of the functional importance of classification schemes based on anatomy, immunocytochemisty, and intrinsic electrophysiological properties. Interestingly, recent results (Simon et al., 2005) indicate that neurogliaform cells (see below), unlike other interneurons, participate in both homologous (with other neurogliaform cells) and heterologous networks (with several other interneuron classes) through electrical synapses. Therefore, neurogliaform cells may link multiple homologous networks formed by gap junctions restricted to a particular class of interneuron.

6. The discovery of the back-projection cell (Sik et al., 1994), an interneuronal species that projects across traditional hippocampal areal boundaries over long distances. The cell body of the back-projection cell was located in the CA1 stratum oriens and it sent its axons all the way to the dentate hilus (Sik et al., 1994). Subsequently, other long-range, cross-areal interneuronal species have also been found, for example, the hippocampo-septal cells (Toth & Freund, 1992; Toth et al., 1993; Gulyás et al., 2003) and interneurons that project from the outer molecular layer of the dentate gyrus to the subiculum (Ceranik et al., 1997), connecting the input and output areas of the hippocampal formation. The existence of interneurons that cross area-specific boundaries is thought to be especially important, as it indicates that extremely long-range connections can originate from dedicated interneuronal species, which, albeit of rare abundance, are predicted to serve crucially important functions in connection with the small world nature of cortical neuronal networks (discussed later in the book).

7. Prediction and subsequent verification of the existence of dendritically projecting CCK-positive interneurons in the hippocampus. The successful search for an interneuronal species that was predicted to exist is an especially clear example of the power of microcircuitry-based, functional anatomical thinking. In the neocortex (as well as other nonhippocampal cortical areas, collectively referred to as isocortex), there are two types of CCK-positive interneurons, the basket cells that innervate the somata and proximal

dendrites, and double bouquet cells that target distal dendrites and dendritic spines. However, in the hippocampus, CCK had only been reported in basket cells, until a study set out to test the prediction that there should be a hippocampal equivalent of the CCK-positive, cortical double bouquet cells. The prediction turned out to be correct, and a hippocampal interneuronal species (the Schaffer-collateral associated interneurons; see also Vida et al., 1998), which proved to be a homologue of the isocortical double bouquet cells, was indeed found and identified (Cope et al., 2002).

8. Discovery of an interneuron species that can generate unitary $GABA_A$ and $GABA_B$ receptor–mediated slow post-synaptic events in its target cells in the neocortex (Tamas et al., 2003), in contrast to all other interneurons that generate exclusively $GABA_A$ receptor–mediated fast unitary events. The slow IPSP-eliciting interneuronal species turned out to be the neurogliaform cell, also described by Cajal as arachniform cells, based on its characteristic, tightly intertwined, unmyelinated local axon ramification (DeFelipe & Jones, 1988; see also Valverde, 1971; Jones, 1975; Kisvarday et al., 1990; Hestrin & Armstrong, 1996; Kawaguchi & Kubota, 1997). These cells have recently been also described in the hippocampus (Price et al., 2005).

The Janus-Face of Order and Variability, and the Dangers of Typology

However powerful is the idea that the brain is not unlike a machine that is made up of a certain number of identifiable cellular parts, it suffers from a rather obvious, frequently encountered yet rarely appreciated, and certainly not fully understood, problem. Namely, unlike a particular machine part which can be manufactured with high precision in large quantities with negligible variability, individuals belonging to a particular, real interneuronal subtype within a neuronal circuit are not exactly the same, as neurons, like most biological entities classified as belonging to the same group, differ from each other to some extent. The degree of difference may appear to be considerable, or it may be insignificant, depending on the methods of measurement and the researchers' point of view. Such differences may exist in details of their axonal and dendritic trees, degrees of ion channel and neurotransmitter receptor expressions, and in many other factors. Most often, this variability is treated as an annoyance at best, and it is frequently "averaged out" in practice, without an analysis of the degree of the cell-to-cell variance within a particular interneuronal population. The loss of cellular variability from our thinking is also aided by representations of interneuronal cell types by their generalized, "averaged" forms. Representing an interneuronal species by its averaged form is an accepted practice that can be extremely useful, because idealization and generalization can help to distill the essence of a particular cell type, which, in turn, can aid in inserting the idealized interneuronal species into its precisely defined "niche" within the microcircuit. However, as we shall argue throughout this book, while the idealization of interneuronal types has been, and continues to be, a valid approach, uncritical "typological thinking" (Mayr, 1982) has its own serious dangers and downsides.

Specifically, when an idealized form of an interneuronal type is inserted into a circuit without any consideration of cell-to-cell variability within that particular interneuronal species, reality is not fully represented. This is because reality is a distribution of forms (or, more generally, a distribution of anatomical or physiological properties), and it is replaced with a typical, or an average version. Again, it is important to emphasize that such a "typological" representation may be appropriate for some purposes, but one should not forget that the averaged form cannot tell the whole story. To use an analogy, one can represent a particular finch species with its idealized form if the goal is to study the graph of the food web of a Galápagos Islands, dismissing the individual differences as irrelevant. However, the variation in beak sizes among the individual finches is a crucial factor that determines how individual finches manage to participate in the food web, and, ultimately, that variation also underlies the evolution of Darwin's finches (Weiner, 1994).

In subsequent chapters, we will show that the "typological thinking" that Mayr (1982) was warning biologists about has serious implications for interneuronal microcircuit research as well. First, when we focus on the idealized form, we can lose sight of the fact that there is, without question, some cell-to-cell variability among individual neurons within a single interneuronal species. Second, we will show that the objectively existing cell-to-cell variability among individual neurons belonging to a single interneuronal species can strongly influence how a network responds to incoming inputs and what types of spontaneous oscillatory behaviors it can display. Third, we will also demonstrate that there are real dangers in trying to represent a cell type by its "averaged" version, and we will also highlight the reasons underlying these dangers. Specifically, we will show, using some crucially important and insightful recent results from the work of Eve Marder and her colleagues, that the "averaged" neuron does not necessarily behave like the individual neurons from which the average was created.

Back to the Future: Early Notions on Variability

Let's briefly address how earlier neuroscientific thinkers, and particularly Cajal, dealt with the conjoint problems of the idealization of cell types and the existence of cell-to-cell variability. This point is especially important in light of the popular notion (e.g., Jacobson, 1993) that Cajal's drawings represent idealized cells that he never actually saw through the microscope. Luckily, a number of Cajal's microscopic slides have been preserved, in which the Golgi-stained neurons are still visible in all their details, and a camera lucida apparatus has been identified among Cajal's laboratory equipment (see chapter 1 in DeFelipe and Jones, 1988). Through some ingenious historical detective work, Edward G. Jones and Javier DeFelipe managed to identify, in several instances, the actual cell that Cajal drew for a particular figure (DeFelipe & Jones, 1988). Thanks to their efforts, "the commonly heard myth, which probably owes its origin to Penfield's introductory note to the English translation of *Neuronismo o Reticularismo* (Cajal, 1954), of Cajal drawing his cells from memory in bed while spattering the wall with ink and wiping his pen on the sheets should now be laid to rest" (DeFelipe & Jones, 1988).

Of course, because Cajal's major goal was to arrive at a deeper understanding of network functions through the ordering of the cellular constituents into rational schemes, it is not surprising that he did not overemphasize the naturally occurring variability in form displayed by his individual Golgi-stained neuronal specimens. Nevertheless, Cajal did point out the existence of variations in the morphology of a particular cell type, its deviations from the "idealized" cell type. For example, in his drawings Cajal often displayed the

variable number and/or positioning of terminals that individual basket cells give to different postsynaptic cells of the same type, even if
he did not place a lot of emphasis on such variability. In describing
the pericellular baskets in the human cerebral cortex, Cajal empha-
sizes the variations in what we would today call postsynaptic target
distributions of basket cell axons (Fig. 1.7) (Cajal, 1899; DeFelipe &
Jones, 1988): "In certain cells, the perisomatic plexus is prolonged
for a certain distance along the apical shaft and basal dendrites . . .
becoming exhausted when it reaches the first bifurcations."

Although Cajal is primarily recognized as a champion of the
"typical," his observations on the nontypical ("in certain cells" in
the above passage), extrasomatic targets of basket cells have also
been fully supported by subsequent research. Combined single-cell
recording and light and electron microscopical experiments from
morphologically and physiologically identified interneurons carried
out from the 1970s (e.g., Gilbert & Wiesel, 1979; Somogyi et al., 1983;
Wiesel & Gilbert, 1983; Kisvárday et al., 1985; Somogyi & Soltesz,
1986; Buhl et al., 1994) showed that neocortical and hippocampal

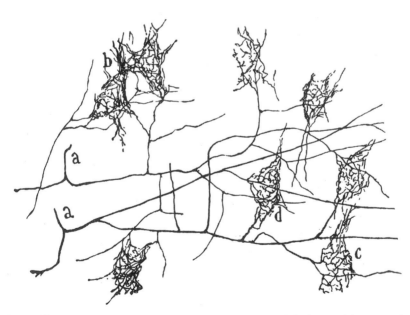

Figure 1.7 **Cajal's drawing of the pericellular arborizations** of the layers of the external
medium and giant pyramids of the motor cortex of the child of 25 days. (a) Axons dividing into long horizontal branches; (b, c, d) pericellular baskets (Cajal, 1899). Reprinted,
with permission, from DeFelipe and Jones (1988).

basket cells frequently innervated the initial portions of the apical dendrites, and they made occasional synapses on axon initial segments as well (more on this later). Furthermore, in spite of the prevailing drive to identify new cell classes and their functional roles, the duality of order and variability has been on the minds of many post-Cajal neuroscientific thinkers. Szentágothai, for example, commented on the apparent duality of order and variability (Szentágothai, 1978; see also Szentágothai & Arbib, 1974; Szentágothai, 1990) this way: "The cortical connectivity is thus a strange mixture between a certain degree of 'randomness' due to the wide spatial distribution of almost all afferent arborizations, and a very high degree of specificity through the micromodular arrangement of the majority of interneurons."

Intriguingly, Szentágothai thought that there was a functional connection between variability and plasticity (Szentágothai, 1978):

This quasi-"randomness" or, to phrase it more carefully, multipotentiality (multi-directionality) of the afferent connections within the boundaries (300 μm in diameter) of the main column, and of the wider non-modular tangential connections in the boundaries of probably 3-6 mm, offers certain potentialities for the so-called plastic properties of the brain. It is a generally accepted notion that there is little room for plasticity of functions in a connectivity system based on a "wiring" that is rigidly predetermined by some blueprint. Conversely, a certain degree of plasticity is intuitively acceptable in a system in which there are inbuilt dynamic possibilities for alternative routes.

As we shall see, these comments on the possible connection between variability and plasticity may turn out to be surprisingly prescient, in the sense that there is now increasing evidence that supports the notion that variability in neuronal connections is an integral, most likely highly regulated property of neural network functions, including plasticity. However, an in-depth attempt at resolving the issue of cell-to-cell variability in identified interneuronal populations was not possible in Szentágothai's time. The field had to await the development of quantitative, higher throughput anatomical, molecular, and physiological methods, as well as advancements in biophysically realistic, large-scale computational network modeling, in order to begin to address the issue of heterogeneity in interneuronal microcircuits in depth.

Defining Interneurons

Before we close this chapter, we should address the thorny issue of what is meant exactly by the term "interneurons." Like most one-word terms that attempt to cover a set of biological entities, the word "interneuron" also has its contentious edges. For example, an earlier term for the cells that are now called interneurons was "local circuit cells." However, as mentioned above, there are now plenty of examples of "interneurons" that project to great distances, often crossing boundaries from one area to the next; for example, from the CA1 region of the hippocampus to the hilus and/or to the septum, or from the dentate molecular layer to the subiculum (Sik et al., 1994; Ceranik et al., 1997; Gulyás et al., 2003). Thus, these neurons cannot be called "local" circuit cells.

A simple definition, especially if we restrict ourselves to cortical networks (and thus excluding several basal ganglia nuclei where GABAergic cells are the numerically dominant projection neurons), is that "cortical interneurons are GABAergic neurons." This latter definition certainly captures the essence of these neurons and is also temptingly concise. However, it suffers from the drawback that it does not address the complex transmitter identity of granule cells in the dentate gyrus. These latter neurons are the principal (in the sense that they are the most numerous) cells in the dentate gyrus, and they normally use glutamate as their primary fast neurotransmitter. However, granule cells clearly have the biochemical machinery to also synthesize and package GABA into vesicles, and they can release GABA (at least in young animals) that can generate inhibitory postsynaptic currents (IPSCs) with relatively slow rise times in CA3 pyramidal cells (Sandler et al. 1991; Lamas et al. 2001; Walker et al., 2001; Gutierrez, 2002). Furthermore, although these cells express only relatively low levels of GABA in normal, healthy situations, their GABAergic phenotype intensifies, both in terms of biochemistry and physiology, following seizures or repetitive stimulations (Schwarzer & Sperk, 1995; Lehmann et al., 1996; Sloviter et al., 1996; Gutierrez & Heinemann, 2001; Ramirez & Gutierrez, 2001; Mody, 2002). In addition to the issue of dentate granule cells, certain texts use the term "interneuron" to include the glutamatergic spiny stellates in the neocortex; however, we regard these latter cells (and other "local circuit" glutamatergic cells, such as the mossy cells of the dentate hilus) as being distinct from the (at least according to our nomenclature) invariably GABAergic interneurons.

Taking some of these issues into account, a slightly more precise definition for a cortical interneuron may be as follows: "A cortical interneuron is a neuron that, in its normal, non-pathological state, uses GABA as its primary fast neurotransmitter." This definition implies that GABA is synthesized in the cell, packaged into vesicles, and, upon its release, binds to GABA receptors present at the majority of its output synapses. Admittedly, this definition is only slightly more satisfying than the simple definition that "cortical interneurons are GABAergic cells" and is also not entirely without holes. For example, there is evidence that some GABA synapses can become "silent" under several conditions (e.g., during low-frequency discharges in certain types of CCK cells in the CA3 region, whose terminals are "muted" by tonically active CB1 receptors; Losonczy et al., 2004; or after barbiturate withdrawal in the CA1 region; Poisbeau et al., 1997). Another issue is that extrasynaptic GABA receptors clearly play an important role in neuronal functions, although the above definition does not exclude that, in addition to intrasynaptic GABA receptors, extrasynaptic GABA receptors also bind the synaptically released GABA (Brickley et al., 1996; Nusser & Soltesz, 2001; Mody & Pearce, 2004). The important issue here is clearly not that we come up with a bulletproof definition but that we agree what we mean by the term "interneuron." The above-stated definition seems to capture the essence of what most interneuron researchers mean by the term cortical "interneurons" today.

2

Developmental Origins of Interneuronal Heterogeneity

> *... all nerve cells when they originate possess essentially the same function ... [the development of their final form] depends solely on the many external influences or stimuli which affect them, and the many possibilities for responding to those stimuli.*
>
> Albrecht von Kölliker (1896)

Ontogenetic Differences between Glutamatergic Neurons versus Interneurons

The fundamental duality of interneuronal subtype diversity on the one hand, and the variance between individual cells belonging to the same subtype on the other, is likely to have its origins in the complex spatiotemporal factors that underlie interneuronal development. The roots of the Janus-faced nature of the order and variance of interneuronal heterogeneity can be traced to two major developmental processes. First, as we shall discuss below in detail, it appears that, right from the time of birth of the postmitotic cells, there is a strict segregation between different cortical cell types in terms of their exact area of origin, both considering glutamatergic cells versus interneurons as a whole, as well as regarding the different interneuronal subtypes. On the other hand, because of the temporal and spatial characteristics of interneuronal migrations, interneurons belonging to the same subtype are likely to experience subtle variations in their ontogenetic histories during their journey from their birthplace to their final positions in the various cortical areas and layers.

Let's first consider the differences between the development of glutamatergic cells and interneurons. The early differences concern several important aspects of their development, including their places of birth and the mechanisms and routes of migration from the proliferative areas to their final destination. Cortical glutamatergic cells originate from the proliferative ventricular zone of the dorsal telencephalon (Sidman & Rakic, 1973). The newly born glutamatergic cells migrate radially from the ventricular zone to the cortical plate, where they form columns of neurons that originate at the same place (Rakic, 1972). The radial migration of neurons, in which cells migrate toward the surface of the brain from the deeper progenitor zones, follows the fundamentally radial design of the neural tube. The process of radial migration is aided by radially arranged glial cells whose processes extend from the proliferative ventricular zone of the neural tube to the pial surface. The distribution of the neurons is according to an inside-out rule, where the early generated neurons form deeper layers, and the subsequently generated cells occupy successively more superficial positions (Rakic, 1988).

In contrast to the glutamatergic cells that are generated locally in proliferative zones deep within the developing cortex near the ventricular wall and migrate radially to their final positions, GABAergic interneurons originate from distant subcortical areas. In a sense, the process of migration and integration of interneurons into the developing cortical areas is reminiscent of the colonization of recently emerged, not yet fully inhabited volcanic oceanic islands by animal and plant species. Getting back to neurobiology, evidence from several species, including humans, indicates that many cortical interneurons derive from the ventral telencephalon in the primordium of the basal ganglia. Figure 2.1 illustrates the location of the various proliferative areas that give rise to interneurons in the developing embryo. The telencephalic vesicles evaginate from the dorsal part of the rostral diencephalons. There are two parts to the telencephalon: the pallium (roof) and the subpallium (base) (Fig. 2.1A). The cerebral cortex and the hippocampus develop from the pallium, whereas the striatal, pallidal, and telencephalic stalk regions compose the subpallium (Marin & Rubenstein, 2003). The embryonic subpallium is the site of origin for what appears to be the vast majority of interneurons in the cerebral cortex and hippocampus (Anderson et al., 1997). Although there are multiple origins for interneurons within the subpallium (see below), most GABAergic interneurons derive from the medial ganglionic eminence (Fig.

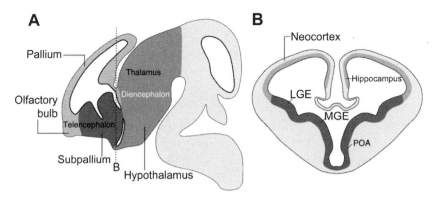

Figure 2.1 **Anatomical organization of the developing forebrain**. (A) Schema of a sagittal section through the brain of an E12.5 mouse showing the main subdivisions of the forebrain, the diencephalon, and the telencephalon. In the telencephalon, the pallium is depicted in lighter gray than the subpallium. (B) Schema of a transversal section through the telencephalon of an E12.5 mouse, indicating some of its main subdivisions. LGE, lateral ganglionic eminence; MGE, medial ganglionic eminence; POA, anterior preoptic area. Reprinted, with permission, from Marin and Rubenstein (2003).

2.1B). The newly generated interneurons have to travel long distances from the subpallium to the cerebral cortex and hippocampus in a manner that, given the nature of the physical relationship between the subpallial proliferative areas and the pallial target zones, has to differ from the simpler radial migration performed by the cortical glutamatergic cells. The interneuronal migration is orthogonal to the direction of the radial migration and is referred to as tangential migration (as the name suggests, one can think of tangential migration as taking place roughly parallel to the pial surface).

Interneurons migrating toward the cerebral cortex and hippocampus appear to follow highly specified avenues. The cortex-bound interneurons, especially during the early stages of their migration, avoid entering the developing striatum (Marin & Rubenstein, 2003). Given their aversion for the striatum, and the fact that the striatal mantle is situated between their birthplace in the medial ganglionic eminence and their final cortical destination, interneurons fated to migrate to the cortex have no choice but to go around the embryonic striatum either via a superficial or a deeper pathway. The superficially migrating cortex-bound interneurons at first do not enter the cortical plate; they migrate in the marginal zone or through the subplate. (Note that, in the embryonic cortex, the first wave of neurons, including the pioneer Cajal–Retzius cells, that migrates radially out of the ventricular zone constitutes the pre-plate, and the second cohort of migrating cells forms the cortical plate, which separates the preplate into two layers: the marginal zone and the subplate.) In contrast, the deeply migrating interneurons initially travel through the lower intermediate zone, and, as develop-ment progresses, these cells occupy a deeper position in the embry-onic cortex, overlapping with the subventricular zone.

In addition to differences in the routes they take around the stria-tum, the interneurons participating in these two migratory path-ways seem to also differ in their preferences for solo versus group travel. Specifically, interneurons that migrate through the marginal zone and subplate tend to travel individually, whereas interneurons that invade the cortical subventricular zone migrate as a compact cluster (Marin & Rubenstein, 2003). Exactly what interneuronal subtypes participate in these two migratory pathways is not yet well understood, but the existence of different migratory streams is likely to further increase the differential array of molecular factors that the distinct interneuronal clusters are exposed to during their development.

Molecular Carrots and Sticks for Interneuronal Migration

Neurons, not unlike humans, need at least three conditions for migration: a reason to leave their current place of residence; a means of transportation, including roads to travel on; and a guidance mech-anism that leads them to their destination. Why do interneurons leave their place of birth in the ganglionic eminence, what kind of molecular and cellular highways do they use in their journey, and how do they find their way to the cortex? Molecules that strongly modulate the migration of projection neurons, such as cyclin-dependent kinase 5 (Cdk5), do not alter the tangential migration of interneurons from the ganglionic eminences to the embryonic cor-tex (Gilmore & Herrup, 2001), indicating that interneuronal migra-tion is likely to be under different molecular control than the signals that guide glutamatergic cells during their radial migration.

In general, there are three different types of factors that direct the tangential migration of interneurons (Fig. 2.2). First, there

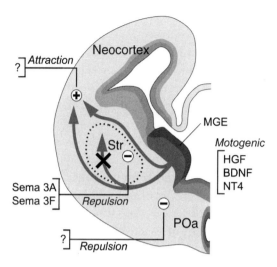

Figure 2.2 **Mechanisms regulating interneuron migration from the subpallium to the cerebral cortex.** Schematic drawing of a transversal section through the telencephalon in which the midline is to the right and dorsal is to the top. (i) Several motogenic factors, including HGF, BDNF, and NT4, promote the migration of neurons from the medial ganglionic eminence (MGE). (ii) An unidentified repulsive activity (*minus sign*) present in the preoptic area (POa) prevents ventral migration of interneurons, directing them toward the cortex. (iii) Expression of Sema3A and Sema3F in the mantle of the developing striatum (Str) prevents cortical interneurons, which express neuropilin receptors, from entering this structure. (iv) An unidentified attractive activity (*plus sign*) guides interneurons toward the cortex and probably contributes to their medial spreading. Reprinted, with permission, from Marin and Rubenstein (2003).

are factors that stimulate interneurons to leave the ganglionic eminences. These "go!" factors are referred to as motogenic factors, and they include hepatocyte growth factor/scatter factor (HGF/SF) (Powell et al., 2001), brain-derived neutrophic factor (BDNF), and neurotrophin-4 (NT4) (Polleux et al., 2001). The observations with HGF/SF are particularly insightful. Antibodies against HGF/SF decrease the number of cells migrating away from the subpallium in slice cultures, whereas HGF/SF itself enhances cell movement. Another way to decrease HGF/SF is to genetically remove the enzyme that converts the inactive proform of HGF/SF to the biologically active protein. Mice lacking such an enzyme, the urokinase-type plasminogen activator receptor (uPar), display a lower number of interneurons at birth than normal mice (Powell et al., 2001).

The second group of factors that is thought to influence the tangential migration of interneurons is the substratum for migration

(Marin & Rubenstein, 2003). Unfortunately, the exact identity of the substratum used by interneurons during their migration has not yet been unequivocally identified. Cortico-fugal axons have been suggested to serve as a potential substratum (Metin et al., 2000; Denaxa et al., 2001), supported by the observation that antibodies against transient axonal glycoprotein-1 (TAG-1) expressed on corticofugal axons reduced the number of interneurons that reached the cortex in slice cultures (Denaxa et al., 2001). However, Tag-1 mutant mice apparently failed to exhibit major alterations in interneuronal migration to the neocortex, and the fact that many migrating cells from the subpallium are concentrated in the lower intermediate zone and in the subventricular zone, both of which contain axons relatively sparsely, also argues against the involvement of axons as primary substrates for interneuronal tangential migration (Marin & Rubenstein, 2003).

In addition to motogenic and substrate-related factors, multiple guidance cues also play important roles by directing the tangentially migrating interneurons to their targets. The ventro-dorsal direction of interneuronal migration appears to be influenced by a chemorepulsive and chemoattractive system in a push–pull fashion (Fig. 2.2). One set of repulsive factors that propel the interneurons from the subpallium to the cortex appears to be generated in the preoptic area, located ventral to the ganglionic eminences. The molecular identity of the chemorepulsive agents derived from the preoptic area has not been clearly determined. Potential candidates include Slits (Zhu et al., 1999), which are large extracellular matrix molecules with chemorepulsive activity for various axons and cells, and Netrin1, which has been suggested to be involved in repelling striatal neurons from the lateral ganglionic eminence (Hamasaki et al., 2001). However, a preoptic area-derived repulsion is still present in mice with mutations in both Slit members expressed in the subpallium, and mice with simultaneous mutations in Slit1, Slit2, and Netrin1 failed to show alterations in the numbers of interneurons (Marin et al., 2003), indicating the existence of additional molecules with chemorepulsive activity influencing interneuronal migration.

Although the nature of the chemorepulsive agents from the preoptic area has not yet been identified, the chemorepulsive molecules underlying the avoidance of the striatum by the cortically bound interneurons are better understood. Here, evidence points to the involvement of the chemorepulsive molecules called class 3 semaphorins, whose repulsive activity is mediated by transmembrane receptors called neuropilins (Raper, 2000; Marin et al., 2001). Interestingly, interneurons that migrate to the cortex express Neuropilin1 and Neuropilin2, whereas inerneurons that invade the striatum do not express these semaphorin receptors, and there is a significant decrease in the number of interneurons in the cortex following disruption of Neuropilin1 and Neuropilin2 functions (Marin et al., 2001).

On the flip side of this molecular push–pull system, there is evidence for the existence of an as-yet unidentified cortical attractive activity for the tangentially migrating interneurons (Marin et al., 2003; Wichterle et al., 2003). Slice-culture experiments showed that the placement of an ectopic cortex next to a developing brain caused a change in the normal migration of interneurons from the medial ganglionic eminence to the embryonic cortex by attracting the migrating cells in a distance-dependent fashion (Marin et al., 2003). Matrigel matrix experiments also demonstrated that cells from the medial ganglionic eminence preferentially migrate toward cortical cells (Marin et al., 2003; Wichterle et al., 2003). Interestingly, this apparently potent cortical attractive activity may be present in a low-lateral to high-medial gradient in the cortex, indicating that it may also serve in the correct dispersion of interneurons among the various cortical areas (Marin & Rubenstein, 2003). A recent study aimed at identifying the attraction signals for cortical interneurons pointed to Neuroregulin-1 and its receptor ErbB4 (Flames et al., 2004). The data showed that the developing cortex and the interneuronal migratory routes expressed isoforms of Neuroregulin-1, whereas ErbB4 was expressed on certain populations of migrating interneurons. Interestingly, the different isoforms of Neuroregulin-1 functioned as short- and long-range attractants, and in vitro or in vivo perturbation of Neuroregulin-1/ErbB signaling decreased the number of migrating interneurons as well as the number of interneurons in the postnatal cortex (Flames et al., 2004).

Distinct Interneurons from Different Sources?

Exactly how many distinct areas serve as the calfing grounds for interneuronal progenitors? Although the medial ganglionic eminence appears to be the primary source of cortical interneurons, several other embryonic brain areas have also been implicated. These secondary areas include the lateral ganglionic eminence, as well as the caudal ganglionic eminence, which is essentially a caudal extension of the fused medial and lateral ganglionic eminences protruding into the lateral ventricle at the level of the mid to caudal thalamus (Xu et al., 2004). In addition, the retrobulbar neuroepithelium of the lateral ventricle (located in the ventrolateral wall of the lateral ventricle rostral to the septal area and just caudal to the olfactory bulb) may also contribute to the cortical interneuronal population (Meyer et al., 1998; Ang et al., 2003), and there are reports indicating that, at least in humans, interneurons may also originate from the cortex itself (Letinic et al., 2002; Rakic & Zecevic, 2003).

How does interneuronal specification take place in these various areas that contribute to the cortical interneuronal pool? Given the multiple sources of origin, the fundamental question is whether distinct interneuronal species derive form distinct areas. Does each proliferative zone give rise to all or many interneuronal subtypes, or are different interneuronal species born in different places?

There is now strong evidence that, just as the glutamatergic and GABAergic cells originate from distinct areas (cortical versus subcortical), there are also spatially separate origins for many of the different interneuronal subtypes. First, fate-mapping experiments in vivo indicated that, unlike calretinin-expressing interneurons, the parvalbumin- and somatostatin-expressing interneurons originate from the medial ganglionic eminence (Wichterle et al., 2001; Anderson et al., 2002; Valcanis & Tan, 2003). Second, in vitro assays, where cells from various telencephalic proliferative zones from green fluorescent protein-expressing (GFP$^+$) donor mouse embryos were transplanted onto neonatal cortical feeder cells in order to determine their ability to generate the various interneuronal species, also showed that parvalbumin- and somatostatin-positive interneurons derive primarily from the medial ganglionic eminence, whereas calretinin-containing interneurons originate mainly from the caudal ganglionic eminence (Xu et al., 2004). Therefore, there seems to be a strict segregation, at least for cortical parvalbumin and somatostatin cells versus calretinin cells, in terms of places of origin.

Regarding the other proliferative areas, the picture is less clear. For example, the lateral ganglionic eminence appears to give rise to striatal medium spiny neurons (Deacon et al., 1994; Stenman et al., 2003), which are GABAergic projection cells expressing the dopamine- and cAMP-regulated neuronal phosphoprotein DARPP32 (Anderson & Reiner, 1991; Xu et al., 2004). In addition, there is evidence that the lateral ganglionic eminence also gives rise to cortical interneurons, although the exact nature of the interneuronal subtypes that derive from the lateral ganglionic eminence is not yet fully established. It appears that the medial ganglionic eminence matures earlier than the lateral one, and the migration from the lateral ganglionic eminence to the cortex is primarily restricted to the later stages of neurogenesis (Anderson et al., 2001). Therefore, there is a difference between the timing of the production of cortical interneurons in the two ganglionic eminences, and there are also differences regarding the precise migratory routes for interneurons that derive from the medial versus the lateral ganglionic eminence (Anderson et al., 2001).

The primary role in the generation of cortical interneurons for the medial ganglionic eminence was also supported by the finding that in the Nkx2.1 mutant mouse, where there is no morphologically distinct medial ganglionic eminence, the somatostatin-positive as well as the parvalbumin-expressing interneuronal subtypes are missing from the cortices (Anderson et al., 2001; Xu et al., 2004). Interestingly, the Nkx2.1 mutants maintain normal migration from the lateral ganglionic eminence (Anderson et al., 2001). These results indicate a causal link between the transcriptional factor Nkx2.1 and the speciation of interneurons. Although it is likely that the transcriptional code for the specification of the various interneuronal subgroups will turn out to be complex, the findings related to Nkx2.1 already pinpoints both some of the upstream processes (such as the homeodomain gene Six3, which confers the ability of the neural tissue to express Nkx2.1), as well as the downstream targets (e.g., the lim-homeodomain genes Lhx6 and Lhx7/8) (Ericson et al., 1995; Shimamura et al., 1995; Kohtz et al., 1998; Sussel et al., 1999; Zhao et al., 2003). It is highly likely that we will see more interesting discoveries relating to the segregated origins of interneuronal subtypes in the near future, both in terms of areas of origin as well as the molecular underpinning of the determination of distinct interneuronal cell fates.

A Case Study: Migration of Interneurons Toward the Hippocampus

Recent data on prenatal interneuronal development in the hippocampus provide an excellent opportunity to summarize and highlight the major features of the above findings. In a series of clever experiments, Pleasure and colleagues (2000) used genetic disruption of embryonic differentiation to obtain strong evidence that hippocampal interneurons derived from the ganglionic eminences and that specific hippocampal interneuronal subtypes originated from distinct subcortical progenitor zones. Evidence from the neocortex, as mentioned above, indicated that the medial and lateral ganglionic eminences contribute substantially to neocortical GABAergic cell populations. The crucial data in support of this latter conclusion were obtained from mice with mutations in Dlx1 and Dlx2 homeobox genes that resulted in defects in the development of both the medial and the lateral ganglionic eminences. Mice with loss of Dlx1/2 homeobox functions had a great (about 75%) reduction in the number of GABAergic cells in the neocortex on the day of birth (Anderson et al., 1997). On the other hand, one can take advantage of the Nkx2.1 mutant mice, in which only the medial ganglionic eminence is affected, to investigate the relative contribution of the medial and lateral ganglionic eminences. In mice with mutations in the Nkx2.1 gene, there is an apparent conversion of the medial ganglionic eminence to a lateral-like phenotype. In the Nkx2.1 mutants, there is an approximately 50% reduction of neocortical interneurons (Sussel et al., 1999), suggesting that the medial ganglionic eminence contributes at least half of the GABAergic cells of the neocortex. Essentially similar approaches, based on the complementary examination of Dlx1/2 and the Nkx2.1 mutants, could be therefore employed to study hippocampal interneurons (Pleasure et al., 2000). Hippocampal interneuron birth reaches is peak at E12.5 (Soriano et al., 1986), and DLX2 could be detected by E15.5 in the hippocampal primordium, but not earlier (note that most DLX^+ cells are GABAergic; Anderson et al., 1997, 1999). When DiI (a fluorescent dye that can be taken up by cells) crystals were placed in the basal telencephalon of coronal sections from E13.5 wild-type mice, fluorescent cells could be detected in the developing hippocampus after 72 hours. In order to provide further evidence for the GABAergic nature of the subcortical cells, E12.5 donor slices were labeled with

BrdU (a substance that labels newly born cells), and the medial ganglionic eminence from a donor slice was transplanted into the medial ganglionic eminence of an E12.5 host slice and cultured for 72 hours. A large percentage of the BrdU-labeled cells in the hippocampus were GABAergic, indicating that many interneurons born on E12.5 migrated to the hippocampal primordium. These experiments, however, could not provide any precise information as to the exact percent of the GABAergic cells in the hippocampus that migrated from the medial ganglionic eminence versus alternative sources. And this is where the Dlx1/2 mutants proved themselves to be extremely informative (again). Astonishingly, there were no GABA$^+$ hippocampal cells in the Dlx1/2 mutants (Pleasure et al., 2000), demonstrating that DLX1/2 function is required for the generation of hippocampal interneurons (in contrast to the complete loss of interneurons from the hippocampus, as mentioned above, Dlx1/2 mutants do show some GABAergic cells in the neocortex). The loss of hippocampal GABAergic cells in these mice took place without any obvious defects in the organization and number of glutamatergic cell layers, suggesting that glutamatergic and GABAergic neurons, at least to some extent, have quite distinct developmental histories. In contrast to the Dlx1/2 mutants, the Nkx2.1 mutant mice, as discussed above, showed a less severe decrease in the number of hippocampal interneurons (about 50%). Although the fate of other cell types is not exactly clear (due to the fact that many interneuronal markers, including parvalbumin, begin to be expressed during the first postnatal week, and the Nkx2.1 mutants display early postnatal lethality), the experiments revealed that the neuropeptide-Y (NPY) and somatostatin-expressing interneuronal populations were missing from the Nkx2.1 mutants, indicating that these NPY/somatostatin-expressing specific subpopulations of hippocampal interneurons are derived from the medial ganglionic eminence.

Taken together, these data suggest that hippocampal interneurons depend on the Dlx1/2 function in the developing basal ganglia (Fig. 2.3), and that the medial ganglionic eminence produces distinct subtypes of hippocampal interneurons. It is not entirely clear why the hippocampal interneuronal populations were more severely affected than the neocortical ones. One idea is that perhaps there are some neocortex-specific GABAergic cells, or, perhaps more likely, the Dlx1/2 mutants may have a not fully penetrant migration defect, and it is simply the longer distance to the hippocampus that underlies the more severe effects. It is interesting to point out here that Dlx genes regulate not only migration but also differentiation of the GABAergic phenotype. As mentioned above, most DLX$^+$ cells are GABAergic (Anderson et al., 1997, 1999), and it appears that most, perhaps all, GABAergic cells express Dlx genes at some point in their development (Pleasure et al., 2000). Furthermore, the close association of the Dlx genes and the interneuronal phenotype is also indicated by the finding that ectopic expression of DLX2 in cortical cells can induce them to produce GABA (Anderson et al., 1999). In addition, recent results suggest that Dlx1 function is actually required for the survival of calretinin-, NPY- and somatostatin-expressing cortical interneurons in the adult (Cobos et al., 2005; Wonder & Anderson, 2005).

Long Road to Tipperary: Consequences of Distant Progenitor Zones for Interneuronal Specification

Based on the available evidence discussed so far, it seems likely that interneurons at the time of starting their migration already belong to fairly distinct subgroups. The fact that interneurons have to cover considerable distances during their migrations is likely to have consequences for the intra-subtype (i.e., cell-to-cell) variance. During the long migration that covers large distances, individual cells belonging to specific interneuronal populations are likely to be subjected to slightly different gradients of the molecular attractant and repulsive factors discussed above. In addition to the three classes of factors (motogenic, substrate-related, and attractant-repulsive signals) that influence tangential migration, the movement of interneurons from the ganglionic eminences toward the cortex may also be influenced by neuronal activity. Tangentially migrating cells can respond with changes in intracellular calcium signals to exogenously applied glutamate and GABA through their N-methyl-D-aspartate (NMDA), alpha-amino-3-hydroxy-5-methyl-4-isoxazole propionic acid (AMPA)/Kainate, and GABA$_A$ receptors on their surface membranes (Metin et al., 2000; Soria & Valdeolmillos, 2002). Although the in situ importance of the endogenously released neurotransmitters is not yet known, glutamate may be released from corticofugal fibers in an activity-dependent manner, and stimulation of AMPA receptors in cultures can cause GABA-release in tangentially

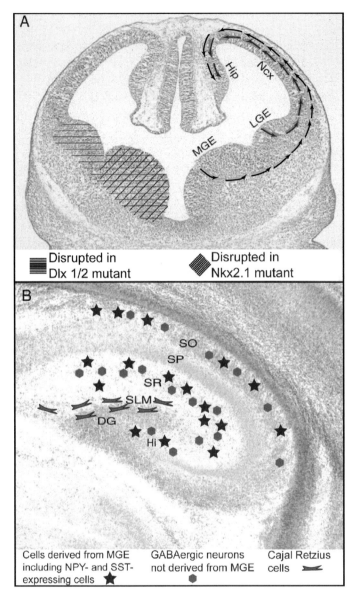

Figure 2.3 **Schematic model of the origin of hippocampal GABAergic interneurons.** (A) E12.5 mouse coronal section stained with Cresyl violet and overlayed with arrows on the right indicating the migratory pathway of cells from the LGE and MGE to the hippocampal anlage. On the left, the regions disrupted by either the Dlx1/2 or Nkx2.1 mutations are indicated by horizontal and slanted cross-hatching, respectively. (B) E19 mouse coronal section stained with Cresyl violet and overlayed with cells of different symbols representing two distinct groups of GABAergic interneurons and Cajal–Retzius cells. LGE, lateral ganglionic eminence; MGE, medial ganglionic eminence; Ncx, neocortex; Hip, hippocampus; Hi, hilus; DGC, dentate granule cell layer; SLM, stratum lacunosum moleculare; SO, stratum oriens; SP, stratum pyramidale; SR, stratum radiatum. Reprinted, with permission, from Pleasure et al. (2000).

migrating cells. The changes in calcium levels resulting from the activity-dependent release of neurotransmitters are potentially significant, as they may lead to a variety of functional and structural alterations in embryonic, developing neurons. Again, individual cells belonging to distinct subclasses are likely to experience differences in the levels of neurotransmitters that they happen to be exposed to during their migration.

As mentioned above, upon arrival in the cortex, the migration of interneurons is not yet finished, as they have to take their position in the proper cell layer in the appropriate cortical area. Therefore, interneurons first undergo tangential migration, then radial migration, following complex trajectories including the diving into the ventricular zone (Marin & Rubenstein 2003). In the end, interneurons seem to follow the same inside-out rule, simultaneously with glutamatergic cells destined to the same layer. During their intracortical migratory phase, local, not yet fully identified cues may also play a role in the fine-tuning of interneuronal phenotypes (Anderson et al., 2001). Therefore, although cortical interneurons seem to be born in specific areas according to their phenotypes, they are exposed to a variety of factors that further influence their development. Exactly how these complex factors interact during migration is not yet clear, but it seems reasonable to suggest that they not only serve to sharpen interneuronal identity but may also underlie, and perhaps regulate the extent of cell-to-cell intragroup variance in distinct interneuronal populations.

When Things Go Wrong: Interneuron Migrations and Neurological Disorders

The assembly of cortical microcircuits requires precise timing of cell migration and differentiation. Because the cortical interneurons are generated at distant subcortical sites, their generation, specification, and long migration are especially susceptible to disruptions (Santhakumar & Soltesz, 2004). Perinatal insults that are relatively nonspecific in nature, such as focal freezing (Prince & Jacobs, 1998), treatment with certain chemicals (Chevassus-au-Louis et al., 1999; Baraban et al., 2000), and viral infections (Pearce et al., 1996), lead to a variety of changes in GABAergic neurons. However, it is the mutations that affect important developmental genes (such as home-obox genes that are the principal orchestrators in the developmental plan of all metazoans) that have the most widespread effects on the interneuronal system (Sherr, 2003; Anderson et al., 1997). As mentioned above, mice lacking the DLX proteins show marked depletion of GABAergic neurons in the neocortex (Anderson et al., 1997) and the hippocampus (Pleasure et al., 2000). Furthermore, mutations in certain homeobox genes (e.g., in the Aristaless Related Homeobox gene) in humans have been found to be associated with severe disorders such as infantile spasms, mental retardation, and autism (Sherr, 2003). In contrast to the widespread effects of home-obox genes, the disruption of genes with more specialized roles in the development of interneurons lead to more region- and subtype-specific changes (Fleck et al., 2000; Powell et al., 2003). For example, disruption of the uPar gene, which, as mentioned previously, is a component in the activation and function of the HGF/SF involved in interneuronal migration, results in a near complete loss of the parvalbumin subtype, with little or no effects on other interneuronal subtypes (Powell et al., 2003). The $uPAR^{-/-}$ mice display enhanced anxiety and spontaneous seizure activity, perhaps as a consequence of diminished interneuronal activity.

Selective modifications in interneuronal populations have also been found in human brain specimens from patients suffering from psychiatric disorders with suspected neurodevelopmental etiology. Results from frontal cortical tissue taken from schizophrenic patients indicate a defective GABAergic system, and there is evidence for a selective decrease in the number of parvalbumin-containing cells (Benes & Berretta, 2001). Whether these data reflect the actual loss of GABAergic cells, or only the decreased expression of markers in the otherwise surviving interneurons (Akbarian et al., 1995), is not yet fully understood. However, recent results that indicate that increased DNA-methyltransferase 1 expression takes place selectively in telencephalic GABAergic neurons in schizophrenic patients may provide interesting insights into the general problem of disease-related alterations in interneuronal markers (Veldic et al., 2004). Specifically, these data suggest that promoter hypermethylation of reelin and glutamic acid decarboxylase-67 (GAD67), and perhaps other genes, may underlie decreased expression of interneuron-specific proteins in these patients (Veldic et al., 2004). Thus, hypermethylation may be a key step in compromising GABAergic function, leading to specific molecular neuropathology and associated functional changes, perhaps not only in schizophrenia but also in other disorders where the loss of specific proteins has been reported from surviving GABAergic neurons (Wittner et al., 2002).

3

Order in Diversity: From Phenomenology to Function

Of all the components that make up the cortical machinery, the most difficult to place has been the GABA-mediated inhibitory system. That is not to say that inhibition is generally thought to be unimportant. On the contrary, inhibition has been used like leaven in bread for every model that requires selective responses from single neurons.

N. Berman, R. Douglas, and K. Martin (1992)

Diversity at Multiple Levels of Neuronal Organization

One of the most interesting aspects of the GABAergic system is its amazing diversity, present at all levels of neuronal organization (in fact, most researchers get "hooked" on interneurons precisely because of their astounding variety). Of course, this extraordinary diversity is also at the heart of many of the technical and conceptual challenges in this field.

At the level of molecules, diversity exists in the form of GABA receptors. There are, to begin with, the Cl^- and bicarbonate-conducting, ionotropic $GABA_A$ receptor-channels, and the K^+- or Ca^{2+}-dependent, metabotropic $GABA_B$ receptors (and a third class, the $GABA_C$ receptors thought to be assembled from ρ-subunits). Within the $GABA_A$ receptor-channel group, there is a large diversity of subunits (e.g., Wisden et al., 1992; Mody, 1995; Hevers & Luddens, 1998). The $GABA_A$ receptor is made up of five subunits (i.e., it is a pentamer), and, given the high number of the currently known sub-unit variants (currently in the high teens, including six α, three β, three γ, one δ, one ϵ, one π, and three ρ), the number of possible combinatorical $GABA_A$ receptors is astronomical. However, the actual, naturally existing diversity is decreased by the fact that only a subset of the possible combinations is used by neurons. Importantly, the different subunit compositions confer distinct functional properties. For example, the presence of a gamma subunit is required for benzodiazepine binding, and the $GABA_A$ receptor contains several distinct receptor sites capable of binding clinically relevant substances such as barbiturates, neurosteroids, and ethanol. A further important aspect of the subunit-dependent diversity comes from the fact that some subunits are preferentially found in receptors that are located outside of the GABA synapses, forming the extrasynaptic receptor pools with interesting, albeit not yet fully understood, functions related to a background GABAergic tone (Brickley et al., 1996; Soltesz & Nusser, 2001; Mody & Pearce, 2004; Farrant & Nusser, 2005). In some cases, receptor subunit diversity can be increased by alternative splicing. Finally, the diversity at the level of the receptors is enhanced even more by the presence of post- versus presynaptic receptors, as is the case for $GABA_B$ receptors.

The second level of diversity in the GABAergic system comes from the existence of different types of interneurons. This is the level of neuronal organization that we already touched upon in earlier chapters, and it will continue to be the primary focus of this book. In order to illustrate the extent of cellular-level order in GABAergic diversity and to discuss the main pillars of modern interneuronal classification schemes, we will list all the known interneuronal species from one cortical area (based on Somogyi & Klausberger, 2005) in the next section.

The GABAergic diversity reflected in the existence of distinct interneuronal cell types can be traced to even higher levels of neuronal organization, to neuronal networks. The best understood of these is the recent discovery, briefly mentioned already in the previous chapter, that distinct interneuronal networks exist as a result of gap junctional, electrical coupling largely restricted to interneurons belonging to the same subtype (Gibson et al., 1999; Galarreta & Hestrin, 1999, 2001; Beierlein et al., 2000; Tamas et al., 2000; Szabadics et al., 2001). For example, fast-spiking (presumed an identified parvalbumin-positive) basket cells tend to be both synaptically and electrically coupled to each other but significantly less to other interneuronal types (Gibson et al., 1999; Galarreta & Hestrin, 1999, 2002; Fukuda & Kosaka, 2000; Tamas et al., 2000). Cannabinoid-receptor containing, presumed CCK-positive cells also innervate each other and may also form gap junctional syncytia (Meyer et al.,

2002; Galarreta et al., 2004). Similarly, preferential gap junctional coupling between relatively homogenous interneuronal populations has been found also between late-spiking cells (Chu et al., 2003), multipolar bursting cells (Blatow et al., 2003), and somatostatin immunopositive or low threshold spiking cells (Gibson et al., 1999; Beierlein et al., 2000; Venance et al., 2000). Interestingly, as mentioned in Chapter 1, neurogliaform cells participate in both homologous and heterologous interneuronal networks through gap junctions (Simon et al., 2005).

Linnean Order in Diversity: A Modern Compendium of Interneuronal Species

Figure 3.1 shows one of the most recent and detailed classification systems for one cortical area, the CA1 region of the hippocampus (Somogyi & Klausberger, 2005). According to this scheme, there are altogether 16 cell types distinguished by a variety of criteria, including the postsynaptic targets (as determined not only by light microscopy but frequently also by electron microscopy), dendritic patterns, and the expression of key immunocytochemical markers. It is an interesting but open question as to exactly how many different interneuronal "species" inhabit just the CA1 region, as it is virtually certain that 16 will not be the final number and that the list is likely to grow longer. In a later chapter, we will come back to this issue and attempt to make an educated guess at the upper limit. We discuss here these 16 interneuronal species in some detail (for more details and full justification of the separation of subtypes, see Somogyi and Klausberger, 2005), because the actual descriptions convey best what the identity of these currently recognized interneuronal subtypes is based on, and these descriptions provide a clean sense of how future work will likely lead to the recognition of additional, separate interneuronal species.

The listing below also indicates that we can delineate at least two major superfamilies of interneurons: one for interneurons that innervate primarily specific domains of pyramidal cells, and one for interneurons that specialize for other interneurons. We will return to the topic of above-species classification units for interneurons later in the book. Some of the cell types were already briefly mentioned in chapter 1, but we will relist them in more details here for the sake of

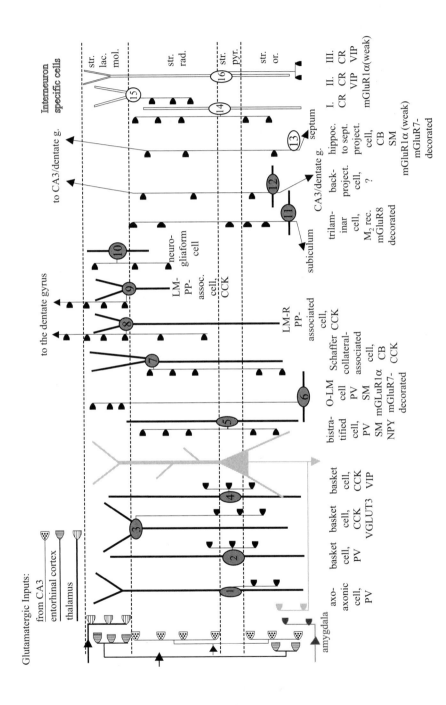

48

Figure 3.1 **Innervation of pyramidal cells by 12 types of GABAergic interneuron and interneurons by 4 types of interneuron-specific cell in the CA1 area of the hippocampus.** The main lamina specific glutamatergic inputs are indicated on the left. The somata and dendrites of interneurons innervating pyramidal cells are shown in gray and black, respectively, and those innervating mainly or exclusively other interneurons are shown in white. The main termination zone of GABAergic synapses are shown by black symbols. The proposed names of neurons, some of them abbreviated, are under each schematic cell and a minimal list of molecular cell markers is given, which in combination with the axonal patterns helps the recognition and characterization of each class. Note that one molecular cell marker may be expressed by several distinct cell types. Some cells are listed on the basis of limited data from one study, and further data may lead to lumping of some classes (see text). Some additional cell types, which have not been reported in sufficient detail, are not indicated. Note the association of the output synapses of different sets of cell types with the perisomatic region and either the Schaffer collateral, commissural, or the entorhinal pathway termination zones, respectively. CB, calbindin; CR, calretinin; LM-PP, lacunosum-moleculare perforant path; LM-R-PP; lacunosum-moleculare radiatum perforant path; M$_2$, muscarinic receptor type 2; NPY, neuropeptide Y; PV, parvalbumin; SM, somatostatin; VGLUT3, vesicular glutamate transporter 3. Adapted, with permission, from Somogyi and Klausberger (2005).

49

completeness. Also note that, in several places, we explicitly noted that the expression of certain key markers are mutually exclusive; for example, a parvalbumin-positive (PV$^+$) cell type is never CCK$^+$, and the reverse is also true; a CCK$^+$ cell that is vasoactive intestinal polypeptide-positive (VIP$^+$) is always negative for vesicular glutamate transporter 3 (VLGUT3$^-$), and vice versa. The 16 interneuronal species currently recognized in the CA1 region are introduced below, like dramatis personae in a *Masterpiece Theater* play, and illustrated in Fig. 3.1, based on Somogyi and Klausberger (2005).

The first 12 species mainly innervate pyramidal cells:

1. **Axo-axonic (chandelier) cells**: These are PV$^+$ cells that innervate excusively (or almost exclusively) the axon initial segments of glutamatergic neurons (in the CA1 region, these are the pyramidal cells; elsewhere in the hippocampus, the targets can be dentate granule cells and hilar mossy cells). The number of postsynaptic target cells is large, a single axo-axonic cell in the CA1 can innervate up to 1,200 pyramidal cells (Somogyi et al., 1983; Li et al., 1992). The GABA released from axo-axonic cell terminals act on α2 subunit containing GABA$_A$ receptors (Buhl et al., 1994b; Nusser et al., 1996; Somogyi et al., 1996). Interestingly, whereas most axo-axonic cells have radial dendrites with an extensive tuft in the stratum lacunosummoleculare, a subset of these cells have been described with exclusively horizontal dendrites (Ganter et al., 2004), which points to the possibility of the future recognition of a functionally separate species. It is also important to recognize that axo-axonic cells frequently cannot be differentiated from basket cells without electron microscopic examination of their target profiles. Also, because there is no exclusive marker for axo-axonic cells, PV positivity alone cannot separate them from the other PV$^+$ cell types, especially from the PV$^+$ basket cells with tight axonal arbor in the pyramidale layer (see below).

2. **PV+ (and thus CCK$^-$) basket cells**: These cells innervate the perisomatic regions (somata and proximal dendrites) of pyramidal cells and other PV$^+$ basket cells (and some other interneurons), and the postsynaptic GABA$_A$ receptors contain the α1 subunit (Buhl et al., 1994a; Ali et al., 1999; Pawelzik et al., 2002). Interestingly, the axonal

arbor can be restricted to the pyramidal cell layer, or it can also occupy to various extents the neighboring radiatum and oriens layers (of course, the proportion of synapses on the dendrites will change accordingly; Pawelzik et al., 2002). The dendrites reach the distal dendritic lacunosum-moleculare layer, but they do not form extensive tufts. These cells are gap-junction coupled (Fukuda & Kosaka, 2000), which, together with the fast kinetics of the interbasket cell IPSCs (Bartos et al., 2002), is thought to aid synchronization.

3. **CCK$^+$ (and thus PV$^-$) basket cells that are VIP$^+$ (and thus VLGUT3$^-$):** The axons are either restricted to the pyramidal cell layer, or they can spread to various degrees to the oriens and radiatum. Consequently, this species innervates the somata and sometimes the proximal dendrites of pyramidal cells (in addition to other CCK$^+$ cells and other interneurons) (Harris et al., 1985; Nunzi et al., 1985). The dendrites enter the lacunosum-moleculare but rarely branch (Pawelzik et al., 2002). The GABA released from the terminals acts on postsynaptic receptors containing primarily the α2 subunit (Thomson et al., 2000; Nyiri et al., 2001).

4. **CCK$^+$ (and thus PV$^-$) basket cells that are VGUT3$^+$ (and thus VIP$^-$):** These cells are similar to type no. 3 above, except for the difference regarding VIP and VGLUT3 immunoreactivity. Because of the VGLUT3 expression, this subtype is listed separately; however, more studies will be needed to determine if the mutually exclusive VIP/VGLUT3 expression patter is related to two states of a single subtype or two genuinely distinct interneuronal species.

5. **Bistratified cells** (Buhl et al., 1994a): These cells are PV$^+$ (and thus CCK$^-$), as well as SOM$^+$ and NPY$^+$, and have high expression of the α1 subunit of the GABA$_A$ receptor on their somatic and dendritic membranes. As mentioned earlier in chapter 1, the axons of these cells are complementary to the classical basket cells, that is, they innervate the oriens and radiatum (but largely avoid the pyramidal cell layer), where they release GABA onto postsynaptic GABA$_A$ receptors (Buhl et al., 1994a; Pawelzik et al., 1999, 2002; Maccaferri et al., 2000) with α5 and γ2 subunits (Pawelzik et al., 1999) on the pyramidal cell

dendrites. These cells also contact basket cells and other interneurons (Halasy et al., 1996; Pawelzik et al., 2003). Similar to the situation with the axo-axonic cells described above, where some cells display distinct (horizontal) dendritic distributions from the classical pattern, there are also reports of some bistratified cells that have horizontal dendrites (Maccaferri et al., 2000), as opposed to the more typical radial distribution. Whether these "oriens-bistratified" cells (Maccaferri et al., 2000) are truly (meaning functionally) different from the bistratified cells will remain to be established.

6. **Oriens to lacunosum-moleculare (OLM) cells**: These are also PV$^+$, albeit their PV immunoreactivity is weaker than it is in the case of previously mentioned PV$^+$ cell types, indicating lower PV expression levels. The cells are also SS$^+$ and strongly mGLUR1α^+, and their glutamatergic and GABAergic presynaptic inputs are distinctively mGLUR7a$^+$ (Shigemoto et al., 1996; Somogyi et al., 2003). The soma and dendrites reside in the oriens, and the majority of the axon is in the lacunosum-moleculare (McBain et al., 1994). They innervate the distal dendrites of pyramidal cells (Maccaferri et al., 2000) and also contact other interneurons (Katona et al., 1999a).

7. **Schaffer-collateral associated (SCA) cell** (Vida et al., 1998): These are CCK$^+$ cells, and at least some are also CB$^+$ (Cope et al., 2002), but they are SOM$^-$ and NPY$^-$. As the name indicates, the axonal projections of these cells overlap with the Schaffer collateral and commissural inputs, where they innervate the apical dendrites (and also the basal dendrites, albeit to a lesser extent), activating postsynaptic GABA$_A$ receptors. It is important to emphasize that the axonal layer specificity is not entirely unlike the axonal distribution of the bistratified cells described above, however, the bistratified cells are PV$^+$ and SOM$^+$, whereas the SCA cells are negative for both. These cells also contact other SCA cells (Pawelzik et al., 2002) and other interneurons (Vida et al., 1998). The dendrites are largely in the radiatum but can also include other layers.

8. **Lacunosum-moleculare–radiatum perforant path–associated cells**: These cells are thought to be CCK$^+$ and CB$^+$,

but the marker-identity of these neurons is not yet fully established. The axons are mainly in the lacunosum-moleculare, with significant spill-over into the radiatum and even the dentate gyrus. Soma is at the lacunosum-radiatum border or in the radiatum, with a wide dedritic field encompassing several layers (Hajos & Mody, 1997; Vida et al., 1998). Clearly, future studies are needed to further delineate the identity of these cells, especially the extent of their separation from the apparently closely related cell type discussed next.

9. **Lacunosum-moleculare perforant path–associated cell**: These cells are also likely to be CCK^+ (Pawelzik et al., 2002), and, as with their cousins discussed above (no. 8), their key immunocytochemical markers also need to be determined further. The axons of these cells are closely associated with the entorhinal input, and it is this feature that is proposed to separate them from type no. 8. It is nevertheless quite possible that types no. 8 and no. 9 may turn out to be members of the same species, and the apparent differences are within the naturally occurring cell-to-cell, intraspecies variance. The axons of type no. 9 can project out of CA1 as well, into the subiculum, pre-subiculum and the dentate gyrus.

10. **Neurogliafom cells**: This is an easily distinguishable species with a caracteristically dense axonal cloud that make synapses on dendrites and spines, and the dendritic fields of these cells are also small and fairly dense (Khazipov et al., 1995; Vida et al., 1998). Neurogliaform cells evoke slow unitary $GABA_A$ and $GABAB_B$ receptor mediated IPSPs (Tamas et al., 2003). A recent study (Price et al., 2005) showed that the majority of hippocampal neurogliaform cells are immunopositive for α-actinin-2 (Ratzliff & Soltesz, 2001) and NPY, and that these cells form extensive cellular networks coupled by $GABA_A/GABA_B$ receptor-mediated chemical and electrical connections with low-pass filter properties.

11. **Trilaminar cells** (Sik et al., 1995): These cells show intense M_2 immunoreactivity on their somata and dendrites, and their presynaptic inputs are intensely $mGluR8a^+$. The key feature of these cells, as their name suggests, is the axonal

distribution, which densely innervates the pyramidale as well as the two neighboring laminae (i.e., the oriens and the radiatum). Their cell bodies and long horizontal dendrites reside in the oriens. This species is thought to project to the subiculum, as well as perhaps to other brain areas.

12. **Back-projection cell** (Sik et al., 1994, 1995): The few known specimens of this species innervate the CA1 and "back-project" to the CA3 and the hilus, hence their name. There is no established immunocytochemical marker for these cells (but they may be NADPH-diaphorase$^+$ and neuronal NO synthase$^+$; Sik et al., 1994). The somata and the horizontal dendrites reside in the oriens layer.

The next four species innervate primarily or exclusively other interneurons:

13. **Hippocampo-septal cells**: These are CB$^+$ and SOM$^+$ cells that project to the septum, as well as to other hippocampal areas, including the CA3 (Gulyás et al., 2003). Their cell bodies with horizontal dendrites are in the oriens, and the intra-CA1 axons can be found in oriens, pyramidale, and radiatum (Zappone & Sloviter, 2001; Jinno & Kosaka, 2002; Gulyás et al., 2003). It was through electron microscopy that the interneuronal nature of their postsynaptic targets was revealed (Gulyás et al., 2003). There is no established marker for these cells, but may show somewhat low levels of mGluR1a expression and may have mGluR7a$^+$ inputs. It should be noted that this species may turn out to be closely related to or perhaps even inseparable from the backprojection cells.

14. **Interneuron-specific cells, type I**: These cells are calretinin-positive (CR$^+$). The axons innervate other CR$^+$ (and CB$^+$) interneurons (Acsády et al., 1996b; Gulyás et al., 1996). Their somata are either in the oriens, pyramidale, or radiatum, and their dendrites extent to most layers.

15. **Interneuron-specific cells, type II**: These cells are VIP$^+$, with axons innervating CCK$^+$/VIP$^+$ basket cells (Acsády et al., 1996b; Gulyás et al., 1996). The somata of these cells are in the radiatum and at the radiatum-lacunosum border,

and the majority of their dendrites are in the lacunosum-moleculare.

16. **Interneuron-specific cells, type III**: These cells are CR^+ and also VIP^+, with their terminals expressing high levels of mGluR7a (Somogyi et al., 2003). The axons innervate primarily the OLM cells (Acsády et al., 1996a; Ferragutiet al., 2004). The somata of these cells are in pyramidale or in the radiatum, and the dendrites can span all layers (Acsády et al., 1996a,b).

From the above list, it is evident that there is a high level of order among the interneurons, in terms of their axonal termination zones and their postsynaptic target specificity, or the expression of immunocytochemical markers. Naturally, this is a still-evolving classification scheme, where future results virtually certain to modify the current compendium. For example, as alluded to above, several of the 16 species may be split into two or more separate species in the future, and, conversely, several currently separate species may be needed to be merged (e.g., some of the last three interneuron-specific cell types).

Cogwheels of Understanding: Functions of Interneuronal Subtypes

What are the functional consequences of the extraordinary, ordered diversity apparent at the levels of molecules, cells, and networks? In the case of GABA receptors, as mentioned above, it is clear that distinct functional roles are indeed conferred by the different subunits of the $GABA_A$ receptor. At the level of cells, the search for specific functional roles for each interneuronal subtype has been pursued vigorously for decades, drawing inspiration from Cajal's vision. The goal of this search has been to assign a function or a set of functions to each well-defined interneuronal cell class in each brain area, with the ultimate goal being a bottom-up description and a virtual (and perhaps one day a physical) assembly of the entire neuronal machine.

The search for assignment of specific functions to interneuronal subtypes has been undertaken using a variety of approaches (Somogyi et al., 1998; Callaway, 2002). Some of the key results came from in vitro slice studies. For example, an important step was the demonstration that dendritically projecting interneurons can effectively regulate Ca^{2+}-spikes, whereas somatically projecting ones are especially effective in modulating the generation of Na^+-spikes (i.e., action potentials) (Miles et al., 1996). In vitro studies also showed that single basket and axo-axonic cells can entrain and synchronize tonicaly discharging pyramidal cells in the hippocampus, through the phase-resetting of intrinsic membrane potential oscillations at the theta frequency (Cobb et al., 1995). Other results reflected how interneurons receive their intrinsic and extrinsic excitatory inputs. Some interneurons, such as OLM cells in CA1, are activated by the CA1 pyramidal cells themselves, and thus function as feedback elements in the circuit. Others, like the cells in the lacunosummoleculare in CA1 that receive direct perforant path input but no CA1 pyramidal cell inputs, seem to be well suited to serve as feed-forward inhibitory elements. In some cases, it was the connectivity to other interneurons that led to insights regarding the functional role of certain interneuronal subtypes. For example, calretinin-positive hippocampal interneurons that exclusively innervate other interneurons (see above; Acsády et al., 1996b; Gulyás et al., 1996) are hypothesized to play a supervisory role in interneuronal networks, perhaps akin to a conductor in an orchestra. It was also in vitro slice recordings that shed light on the neurogliaform cells that evoke $GABA_B$ responses in postsynaptic cells, indicating their preferential involvement in slow inhibition, at least in the neocortex (Tamas et al., 2003).

In addition, combined somatic and dendritic recordings in slices revealed that, during a series of action potential discharges in pyramidal cells, recurrent inhibition rapidly shifts from the somata to the apical dendrites, through the precise, sequential recruitment of two distinct interneuronal circuits (Pouille & Scanziani, 2004). The perisomatically projecting interneurons are recruited during the initial part of a pyramidal cell discharge, causing a transient inhibition of the somatic regions of pyramidal cells. Next, it is the dendritically projecting interneurons that are recruited by the sustained pyramidal cell discharge, resulting in inhibition of the distal apical dendrites. These two operating modes are made possible by tightly regulated, precise differences in short-term plasticity of the excitatory inputs to the two groups of interneurons, in that the pyramidal cell excitation of the perisomatically projecting interneurons shows

prominent depression, whereas the excitatory inputs to the dendritically projecting recurrent interneurons display facilitation (Puille &
Scanziani, 2004).

It is clear that systems-level understanding of the functional roles
of interneurons has to come from in vivo recordings. Here, the
attention has been focused on the relationship of the firing of
certain interneuronal subtypes to synchronized activity patterns in
large principal cell populations taking place at various frequencies.
Single-cell intracellular recordings in anesthetized preparations
revealed that basket cells are major generators of the hippocampal
gamma and theta oscillations (Soltesz & Deschênes, 1993; Ylinen et
al., 1995), indicating that the functional contribution of these
interneurons is much more diverse than previously thought and is
certainly not limited to simple "inhibition" functioning purely as a
brake against overexcitation.

Subsequently, using the technique of juxtacellular in vivo recording in anesthetized rats (Pineault, 1994) that allowed the noninva-
sive, extracellular recording and subsequent visualization of cells,
the discharge patterns of anatomically identified interneuronal subtypes during network rhythms were studied in a much greater detail
in a series of seminal papers (Klausberger et al., 2003, 2004). A key
finding was the recognition that distinct, phase-related firing
patterns (with respect to the extracellularly recorded field activity,
representing the average population activity) of the various interneuronal species in the CA1 region were correlated with the spatial
specificity of the interneuronal axonal outputs. Specifically, these
studies revealed that, during theta activity, axo-axonic cells fire with
the highest probability during the peak of the extracellularly
recorded theta rhythm in the pyramidal cell layer (Fig. 3.2), which
is the phase of the theta oscillations when the pyramidal cell is
the most hyperpolarized. (Actually, the intra- and extracellularly
recorded theta oscillations are not perfectly out of phase: the peak
of the intracellular theta recorded from the somata of pyramidal
cells lags by 0–60 degrees the trough of the extracellular theta in the
pyramidal cell layer [Soltesz & Deschênes, 1993]; the peak of the
intracellular theta recorded in the dendrites of the pyramidal cell
lags the peak of the extracellular theta recorded in the pyramidal
cell layer [Kamondi et al., 1998].) In contrast, PV^+ basket cells fired
slightly after the axo-axonic cells, on the descending phase of the
extracellular theta recorded in the pyramidal cell layer (Fig. 3.2).

Bistratified cells and OLM cells fired at a similar phase after the PV^+ basket cells, during the trough of the extracellular theta reorded in the pyramidal cell layer (Fig. 3.2). Because pyramidal cells tend to fire (albeit at a low rate during theta) when their somata is the most depolarized (during or slightly after the trough of the extracellular theta recorded in the pyramidal cell layer), these data indicate that pyramidal cell firing takes place after the highest firing probability of axo-axonic and basket cells, perhaps indicating the timing and synchronization of pyramidal cell membrane potential oscillations by these interneurons, similar to observations in vitro (Cobb et al., 1995). Curiously, these data also indicated that pyramidal cell firing appeared to be coincident with the maximal firing of the dendritically projecting interneurons, the bistratified cells and OLM cells, when the relative dendritic hyperpolarization is maximal (Klausberger et al., 2003, 2004). It has been suggested that this may be a kind of threshold mechanism that insures that only the strongest inputs result in pyramidal cell firing and may also contribute to various postinhibitory rebound firing phenomena in the dendrites (Somogyi & Klausberger, 2005). In contrast to theta oscillations that occur in unanesthetized, freely moving animals during whole-body movements, various memory tasks and rapid eye movement sleep (Grastyan et al., 1959; Vanderwolf, 1969), sharp wave-associated ripple oscillations (duration: around 100 ms; frequency: 120–200 Hz; initated by the coordinated discharge of a subset of CA3 pyramidal cells) take place in the CA1 region during slow-wave sleep and consummatory behaviors (Buzsáki et al., 1983). During ripples, some (but not all) CA1 pyramidal cells fire one or a few action potentials phased-locked to the trough of the extracellularly recorded ripples. At the same time, PV^+ basket cells and bistratified cells also increased their discharge frequency during the ripple episodes (Fig. 3.2). Interestingly, bistratified cells increased their firing rates even before ripples could be detected on the extracellular trace, and they maintained their high-frequency firing throughout the ripple, whereas basket cells fired most at the highest amplitude ripples (Fig. 3.2). Axo-axonic cells and OLM cells behaved markedly differently from the basket cells and bistratified cells. Axo-axonic cells increased their firing as the ripples began, but they turned silent right after the highest amplitude ripples and stayed silent even after the ripple episode (Fig. 3.2). In contrast, OLM cells appeared suppressed for the entire period of the ripples, perhaps indicating the presence of

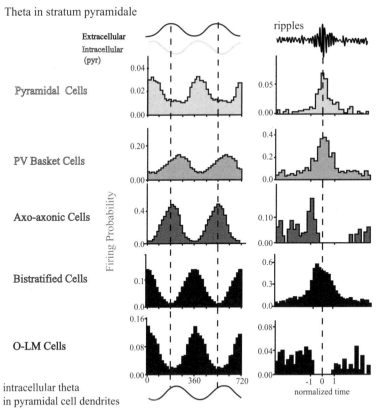

Theta in stratum pyramidale

Pyramidal Cells

PV Basket Cells

Axo-axonic Cells

Bistratified Cells

O-LM Cells

intracellular theta
in pyramidal cell dendrites

Figure 3.2 **Distinct in vivo firing patterns of pyramidal cells and four types of interneuron embedded in the hippocampal network.** The CA1 pyramidal cells, parvalbumin expressing basket, axo-axonic, bistratified, and OLM cells have differential temporal firing patterns during theta and ripple oscillations (mean of several cells). For clarity, two theta cycles are shown in the firing probability histograms. The Y axis of the spike probability plots was constructed by including all events and cycles in the analyzed period irrespective of whether the individual recorded cell fired or not. The phase relationship of the extracellularly recorded field potential (schematic wave) used in the spike alignments and the phase shifted oscillation in the membrane potential oscillation of pyramidal cells reported from intracellular studies is shown schematically. For the ripples, time was normalized to the beginning, highest amplitude and end of ripple episode. The spike probability plots show that during different network oscillations representing two distinct brain states, interneurons of the same connectivity class show different firing activities and therefore modulate their specific postsynaptic target-domain in a brain-state-dependent manner. Interneurons belonging to different connectivity classes fire preferentially at distinct time points during a given oscillation. Because the different interneurons innervate distinct domains of the pyramidal cells, the respective compartments will receive GABAergic input at different time points. This suggests a role for interneurons in the temporal structuring of the activity of pyramidal cells and their inputs via their respective target domain in a cooperative manner, rather than simply providing generalized inhibition. Original versions of the firing probability histograms first appeared in Klausberger et al. (2003, 2004). Adapted, with permission from Somogyi and Klausberger (2005).

inhibitory inputs to OLM cells from other interneurons (Somogyi & Klausberger, 2005).

Taken together, these data indicated the existence of interneuron species-specific firing behaviors during theta and ripple network oscillations. It is important to emphasize here that, in the most general sense, the presence of cell type-specific firing patterns for the various interneuronal subgroups was predictable, and entirely to be expected, from Cajal's research paradigm. Namely, if each interneuronal species, endowed with a specific morphology and a characteristic set of neurotransmitter receptors and ion channels, occupies a specific position in the neuronal network with highly subtype-specific, distinct input–output connectivity, then interneuronal subtypes in a given circuit should behave differently during network oscillatory activities. These data also indicate that, at some point in the future, when our knowledge of the anatomical and physiological properties of the individual interneuronal species reaches a certain point, we should be able to explicitly predict the firing patterns of the various cell types in detailed, large-scale computational simulations incorporating realistic single-cell models and network connectivity rules (Dyhrfjeld-Johnsen et al., 2004; Traub et al., 2005; Santhakumar et al., 2005).

Interestingly, the results on the firing of interneurons in theta-gamma and ripple oscillations in vivo inspired in vitro studies that developed ingenious experimental slice models for the various network activity patterns seen in vivo (Traub et al. 1999; Whittington & Traub, 2003). For example, bath-applied carbachol can evoke persistent gamma oscillations in slices (Fisahn et al., 1998), and various other drugs and manipulations, such as kainate, high potassium, and tetanic stimulation can all result in transient or persistent oscillatory patterns in vitro. Experiments using these novel in vitro paradigms determined that specific patterns of firing exist even in slices for the various interneuronal subtypes during the oscillatory network activities, in general agreement with the in vivo data. During kainate-induced gamma, for example, OLM cells fired intermittently at the theta frequency, basket cells and bistratified cells discharged predominantly single action potentials on every gamma cycle, whereas trilaminar cells also discharged on every gamma cycle but they tended to fire spike doublets (Gloveli et al., 2005). Based on these observations and the anatomical properties of these cells, it has been suggested that OLM cells may provide theta-frequency patterned outputs to distal dendrites; basket and bistratified cells contribute to the local generation of gamma oscillations. The trilaminar cells may then distribute the local gamma to distal sites (Gloveli et al., 2005). Thus, these slice studies supported the notion that a division of labor exists whereby different interneuronal subtypes mediate the different frequencies and spatiotemporal patterns on hippocampal network oscillations (Hajos et al., 2004).

But getting back to the in vivo studies, it should be noted that anesthetized preparations are not entirely ideal, as it is not possible to directly investigate interneurons during actual animal behaviors. The relationship of interneuronal unit activity patterns to EEG and related sleep/wake states has been studied in freely moving animals (Buzsáki et al., 1983; Colom & Bland, 1987; Kodama et al., 1989; Mizumori et al., 1990; Csicsvari et al., 1999), however, the identity of the recorded units could not be determined. Nevertheless, these results revealed that, in anatomically unidentified hippocampal interneurons in conscious rats, similar profiles of activity can be observed during corresponding network states as in the anesthetized preparations (Klausberger et al., 2003, 2004). Our knowledge about the precise firing patterns of specific interneuronal subtypes during species-specific, natural behaviors is still limited, mostly due to the technical difficulties involved in the precise identification of the recorded units. For example, CA1 interneurons as a whole tend to decrease their firing rates as rats foraged in novel compared to familiar environments (Wilson & McNaughton, 1993), but there appeared to be no layer-specific differences between the recorded units that would indicate obvious cell type-specific firing behaviors (Nitz & McNaughton, 2004). Future studies, based on the visualization and unequivocal anatomical identification of the recorded interneuronal extracellular units, are expected to reveal such differences. Even these unidentified unit recordings revealed that, in contrast to CA1 interneurons, dentate gyrus interneurons exhibited large increases in activity in novel environments, indicating that interneuronal networks in these two areas are modulated in a divergent fashion during the incorporation of novel spatial information into the spatial representation of the familiar environment (Nitz & McNaughton, 2004). What is the actual functional role of the changes in interneuronal activity is, of course, a crucial question. One insight into this issue is the observation that whereas CA1 interneurons decreased their activities, principal cells increased their firing rates, an arrangement that perhaps allows synaptic potentiation of afferents to CA1 pyramidal cells to take place and, therefore, the development of new associations between self-motion cues and external landmarks (Nitz & McNaughton, 2004). Independent evidence also indicates that interneuron activity undergoes alterations during spatial learning in exploration tasks (Moser, 1996). Based on paired-pulse data to assess recurrent inhibition in the dentate gyrus, it has been suggested that exploration is coupled to enhanced activity of dendritically projecting interneuronal populations, whereas inhibition in the somata is decreased, presumably as a result of decreased basket cell activity (Moser, 1996). These results indicate that different populations of interneurons may be differentially engaged during specific behaviors.

Recent computational modeling studies also started to contribute in a major way to the understanding of the differential computational functions of interneuronal subtypes in a behavioral context. For example, in a cortical microcircuit model of spatial working memory, distinct subtypes of interneurons appeared to play different roles (Wang et al., 2004). Basket cells produced widespread inhibition leading to the stimulus tuning of persistent activity, whereas localized disinhibition of pyramidal cells arose through the involvement of interneuron-targeting (representing calretinin-containing) interneurons. A key feature of working memory is the resistence against distracting stimuli, which appeared to be controlled by dendrite-targeting interneurons (Wang et al., 2004).

Finally, it should be noted that, without an indication of the level of organization that is used as a point of reference, it is not always obvious what is meant by "functional roles" of a particular interneuronal species. For example, one can talk about interneuronal functions at the level of the local circuit (e.g., "feedback perisomatic inhibition"), or at the level of the network (e.g., phase-specific discharges during theta-gamma oscillations), or at the level of the conscious behavior of the animal (e.g., firing pattern in relationship to a particular behavioral task). Of course, all of these descriptions are valid, but they represent different levels of analysis.

Basket Cells: Division of Labor

By far, the best understood interneurons in terms of their connectivity, physiology, molecular characteristics, as well as the microcircuit-, network-, and even behavioral-level functional roles, are the basket cells in the hippocampus. In the case of basket cell subtypes, there appears to be a clear division of labor in terms of functions. Figure 3.3 shows the structural and molecular segregation that occurs between two distinct basket cell populations. Basket cells are either parvalbumin- or CCK-positive (note that there are PV^+ cells and CCK^+ cells that are not basket cells; see above). The binary expression pattern of parvalbumin or CCK in basket cells seems to determine the expression of a number of other functionally important molecules (for a review, see Freund, 2003). First, intracellular recordings have revealed that PV-containing cells tend to be fast-spiking, nonaccomodating, capable of discharging at frequencies in the excess of 100 Hz, whereas CCK-cells tend to be regular spiking, usually accommodating during repeated discharges, and they have lower maximum firing rates. In addition to differences in firing properties, GABA-release may also be different, due to the differential expression of presynaptic voltage-gated Ca^{2+}-channels. Indirectly identified CCK-cells appeared to express N-type Ca^{2+}-channels, whereas the presumed PV-positive basket cell terminals expressed P/Q-type Ca^{2+}-channels (Wilson et al., 2001). Beyond differences in the expression of voltage-gated channels underlying action potential characteristics and presynaptic voltage-gated Ca^{2+}-channels shaping GABA-release, there is strong evidence indicating differences in presynaptic receptors, postsynaptic actions, and local and subcortical inputs (Fig. 3.3). PV^+ basket cells form synapses on pyramidal cells mostly through the involvement of postsynaptic $GABA_A$ receptors containing the $\alpha 1$ subunit (Thomson et al., 2000; Klausberger et al., 2002), whereas the synapses formed by CCK^+ cells are rich in $\alpha 2$ subunits (Nyiri et al., 2002). Because benzodiazepine-based anxiolytic actions are selectively mediated by $\alpha 2$ subunit–containing $GABA_A$ receptors (Low et al., 2000), it has been suggested that anxiolysis may take place via the selective potentiation of inhibition originating from CCK^+, but not the PV-expressing, interneurons (Freund, 2003). The axon terminals of PV^+ cells are devoid of CB1-receptors, whereas CCK^+ cells express CB1-receptors at high levels (Katona et al., 1999b), which enables postsynaptic target cells to selectively decrease GABA-release from CCK^+ cells, but not from PV^+ cells, via a retrograde mechanism that is thought to involve the activity-dependent synthesis and release of endocannabinoid substances from the postsynaptic cells and the binding of the endocannabinoid ligands to the presynaptic CB1 receptors. Serotonin type-3 (5-HT_3)

receptors, whose antagonists have strong anxiolytic effects, are also preferentially expressed on CCK[+] neurons, but not on PV[+], cells, and the pattern of serotonergic innervation of CCK[+], but not the PV-containing, interneurons perfectly matches the expression of 5-HT$_3$ receptors (Tecott et al., 1993; Morales & Bloom, 1997; Freund et al., 1990; Papp et al., 1999; Ferezou et al., 2002). In addition to differences in the serotonin-containing subcortical afferents and their modulatory effects on CCK[+] versus PV[+] cells, the action of acethylcholine (ACh) also differs on these two basket cell population. CCK[+] cells express the nicotinic receptor subunit α7 (in the hippocampus) (Freedman et al., 1993; Frazier et al., 1998), whereas PV[+] cells express M$_2$-type muscarinic receptors presynaptically (Hajos et al., 1998) (Fig. 3.3). As a result, ACh depolarizes CCK[+] cells (thus enhancing GABAergic inhibition originating from these interneurons), but it reduces the release of GABA from the terminals of PV[+] basket cells. In addition to all of the differences mentioned above, there are differences in local afferent innervation patterns as well. PV[+] cells receive a lot more glutamatergic excitatory drive, whereas the relative weight of inhibition is stronger for CCK[+] cells (Gulyás et al., 1999; Matyas et al., 2004). The glutamatergic innervation differs not only quantitatively but also in the density of NMDA-receptors, whose expression in glutamatergic synapses on PV[+] interneurons is much sparser compared to CCK[+] cells (Nyiri et al., 2003). Finally, the interneuron-selective calretinin-positive cells innervate the CCK[+] cells but not the PV[+] interneurons (Gulyás et al., 1996).

As the above discussion illustrates, there is an abundance of evidence indicating the segregation of molecules and related functional differences between the two basket cell populations. Interestingly, as proposed recently in a new hypothesis (Freund, 2003), there may be an overarching theme to these multiple, seemingly independent differences. Namely, according to the hypothesis, PV[+] basket cells are a kind of rigid, nonplastic precision clockwork, whereas the CCK[+] interneurons would constitute a readily modifiable inhibitory system through which emotional and motivational effects of the serotonergic and cholinergic pathways are exerted (Freund, 2003). Indeed, many of the above-discussed observations seem to follow this logic. PV[+] cells appear to be particularly well-suited to generate precisely timed oscillatory rhythms due to their capacity for fast, nonadaptive firing, and their interconnections through both synaptic and electrical synapses can enhance their abil-

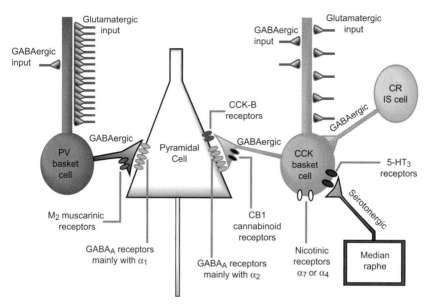

Figure 3.3 **Major differences between parvalbumin (PV)- and cholecystokinin (CCK)-containing basket cells** in their connectivity features and receptor expression patterns. Each axon terminal synapsing on the interneurons (glutamatergic or GABAergic) corresponds to ~1,000 synapses, reflecting true differences in the relative weight of excitatory and inhibitory inputs. CCK-containing cells express presynaptic CB1 cannabinoid receptors and postsynaptic 5-HT$_3$ (5-hydroxytryptamine, serotonin type 3) receptors and nicotinic α7 (or α4) ACh receptors. They receive input from serotonergic median raphe afferents and local interneuron-selective inhibitory cells expressing calretinin (CR IS cell). All of these features are absent in PV-containing cells, but these cells express presynaptic M$_2$ muscarinic receptors. Knowing that anxiolytic effects of benzodiazepines are mediated solely by α2 subunit–containing GABA$_A$ receptors, it is important to note that synapses formed by CCK-positive basket cells on pyramidal cells operate mostly via α2 subunit–containing GABA$_A$ receptors, whereas PV-positive basket-cell synapses contain largely α1 subunits. Adapted, with permission, from Freund (2003).

ity to achieve a high degree of synchrony. CCK$^+$ cells, in contrast, express CB1, 5-HT3, nicotinic receptors, and thus can be the subjects of a variety of modulatory influences. Through the expression of various receptors involved in modulatory actions, CCK$^+$ cells may play a special role in emotional states such as mood and anxiety. The rigid, conservative nature of the PV$^+$ basket cell population may also be reflected in the fact that PV-containing axon terminals are found predominantly within or immediately adjacent to cell body layers. In contrast, CCK$^+$ cells appear to form a continuum, ranging all the way from typical basket cells, through wide-axonal basket cells, to bistratified cells (and other cell types, see above). In summary, according to the hypothesis (Freund, 2003), the molecular segregation is proposed to result in a clear physiological, and even cognitive, division of labor between these two cell types. PV^+ cells are the rhythm-generators, working as the neuronal clocks in the circuit, whereas the CCK^+ cells are the mood-related interneurons, sensitive to the emotional, motivational, and general physiological state. Irrespective of whether or not this hypothesis will survive the test of time, it is inspiring that it is now possible to form specific, data-driven hypotheses regarding distinct patterns of division of labor between specific basket cell types, all the way from molecules to higher cortical functions.

Canonical Microcircuits, Cortical Columns, and Their Stereotyped Inhabitants

If different types of interneurons are specialized to exert specific effects (e.g., on action-potential discharges, dendritic processing, summation of synaptic potentials, or any other potential microcircuit-level functions), it is conceivable that a unit of cortical circuit could be found that would contain all the necessary individual components. Supracellular assemblies of various sizes and types that could serve as cortical units have been the veritable holy grail of microcircuit research for decades. Several designs have been proposed, including the canonical microcircuits, microcolumns, columns, hypercolumns, and the lamellae of the hippocampus (Andersen et al., 1971, 2000; Sur et al., 1980; Amaral & Witter, 1989; Douglas et al., 1989; Bartfeld & Grinvald, 1992; Mountcastle, 1997; Bush & Priebe, 1998; Douglas & Martin, 2004). As far as interneurons are concerned, it appears logical that a "miminal circuit" should contain at least one individual from every interneuronal species, plus one cell representing the principal cell class. In this sense, therefore, the 16 interneuronal species defined above and illustrated in Fig. 3.1, together with a pyramidal cell, could be considered a unit of the CA1 region. Thus, building a model unitary circuit could be imagined to be carried out by inserting a basket cell, an axo-axonic cell, and OLM cell, and so forth, and connecting them in an appropriate, realistic manner to the pyramidal cell and to each other. Once we have our CA1 unitary circuit, with its inputs and outputs, all we need to do is to place a large number of these units in parallel, and establish connections between the units to allow for crosstalk, in order to get a fully functioning CA1 network. The unit can be multiplied many times to get a functional full network, similar to the replication of a basic molecular arrangement resulting in a crystal (although, evidently, such a network would not have the correct ratios of cell numbers for the various subtypes).

Because the unit is multiplied many times, it has to contain idealized, averaged cells. If we chose to include, say, CCK^+ basket cells in our basic unit, the construction of that model cell has to embody the average, typical features of real, biological CCK^+ basket cells determined from experiments. For example, we may measure the mean action potential height, the mean adaptation rates, the mean input resistances, the mean size of the somata, the mean density of various voltage-gated conductances, and the mean of many other parameters. An essentially similar, mean-oriented approach is used in multicompartmental modeling of microcircuits, where the interneuronal subtypes are constructed from the averaged synaptic and voltage-gated conductances measured in experiments (Bartos et al., 2001, 2002; Traub et al., 2004; Wang et al., 2004; Santhakumar et al., 2005). The resulting circuits, in spite of the mean-based approach, are quite successful in replicating the responses of the biological system to pulse activation of the major afferents, and they can also simulate well the effects of the loss of specific cell types and reactive axonal sprouting in neurological diseases (Santhakumar et al., 2004; Dyhfjeld-Johnsen et al., 2004).

If one is not interested primarily in how individual cell types behave or what effect the loss of a particular interneuronal species may have, one can reduce the number of cell types by merging those species that appear to serve overlapping and similar functions in a particular task. How far can one take the merging of species and still have a reasonably well-functioning model network? This question is interesting not only from a theoretical perspective, but also from a practical one, as large networks consisting of multicompartmental single model neurons are complex and computationally intensive, with each conductance being explicitly modeled in each cell in every neuronal subtype. A minimalist approach is embodied in the canonical microcircuit idea, whose inventors, Rodney Douglas and Kevin Martin (Douglas et al., 1989; Douglas & Martin, 1991), used Occam's razor with abandon to shave the number of variables to a minimum, to reduce the number of cell types in the circuit to as much as

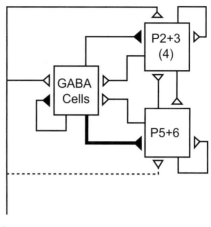

Thalamus

Figure 3.4 **The Canonical Cortical Microcircuit**, circa 1989. Three functional classes of cortical neurons are distinguished: superficial pyramidal cells (P2+3; including also layer 4 spiny stellates), deep layer pyramidal neurons (P5+6), and GABAergic neurons. Some neurons within each population receive excitatory input from the thalamus. Continuous versus dashed lines indicate that thalamic drive to the superficial group is stronger. The inhibitory inputs activate both $GABA_A$ and $GABA_B$ receptors on pyramidal cells. The thick continuous line connecting the GABA neurons to P5+6 indicate that the inhibitory input to the deep pyramidal population is relatively greater than that to the superficial population. However, the increased inhibition is due to enhanced $GABA_A$ drive only. The $GABA_B$ inputs to P5+6 are similar to those applied to P2+3. Adapted, with permission, from Douglas and Martin (1991).

possible (note that "canonical" here is meant in the mathematical sense of simplest, clearest form of microcircuit). For interneurons, the reduction was taken to its limit; that is, the canonical microcircuit has only a single GABAergic interneuron, in addition to two forms of excitatory neurons (Fig. 3.4). What is important from our point of view here is the fact that the behavior of each neuronal population (one interneuron and two excitatory cell types) was modeled by a single neuron that represented the average of neurons belonging to that population (Berman et al., 1992). Therefore, the canonical microcircuit represents the average connectivity and physiology of a patch of cortex. Although the circuit does not differentiate between the different GABAergic neurons, it replicates at least certain types of biological responses surprisingly well. For example, the circuit mimics the appearance of excitatory postsynaptic potentials (EPSPs) and IPSPs in the excitatory cells after a single stimulus pulse applied to the major afferent pathway, and two identical modules of the canonical microcircuit can be linked to simulate directionality in the visual cortex (Berman et al., 1992). Therefore, the approach taken by Douglas and colleagues was to avoid differentiating interneuronal types into functional subgroups until there was a compelling argument to do so. As we saw above, since the conception of the canonical microcircuit idea, there has been an explosion in our understanding of differences between interneuronal species in terms of their possible functional roles in microcircuits. Although the canonical microcircuit provides a clear indication that circuits built from averaged, even merged, neuronal subtypes can perform surprisingly well, at least in certain tests and under specific conditions, it is also likely that many, and perhaps most, distinct interneuronal species would be needed to be represented in realistic models aiming at reproducing realistic network behaviors during complex, behaviorally relevant tasks.

Crusade for the Great Synthesis and the End of Neuroscience

The considerable successes and advancements of the basic paradigm, first outlined by Cajal and pursued by so many excellent minds ever since its conception, define a clear, and one may say inevitable, roadmap for the future of interneuronal research. Namely, we need to finish the identification of all the interneuronal species that exist in any given cortical area to arrive at a complete catalogue of species, we need to determine the exact axo-somato-dendritic position of the various voltage-gated ion channels, neurotransmitter receptors, and second-messenger systems that are differentially expressed among subtypes, and we need to understand how the individual species modulate principal cell discharges, how they interact with each other, and how they behave under various in vivo conditions. In other words, the paradigm first outlined by Cajal needs to be fulfilled and his research program completed. As the necessary empirical data are gathered, we may also build detailed, realistic, biophysically and anatomically accurate computer models for each interneuronal species to deepen our understanding of how they function. For example, through such computer models, we could inactivate individual interneuronal subtypes, in order to assess their roles in both normal and pathological processes. Genetic approaches may also help in determining the effects of cell type–specific deletions on circuit behavior. In a sense, therefore, we see the end of neuroscience, at least as it applies to interneuronal microcircuit research, as we can imagine the complete universe of discoverable facts within the current paradigm. Surprises may be of course plentiful, but the basic nature of the approach, how we piece the new correlations, functional roles, the cellular, receptor, and ion channel subtypes into the preexisting picture, is not expected to be changed. Thus, the roadmap to fulfill the Cajal-paradigm is clear, and the eventual fulfillment of this paradigm can be considered to constitute the great synthesis, the ultimate goal.

The crusade toward the great synthesis continues to produce astonishing testimonies to the crystal-like structure of cortical microcircuits (see Nelson, 2002). Perhaps the best example is the recent report that not only are the cell classes targeted by pyramidal cell axons highly specific, but even the relative positions of the target neurons are precisely defined and subtype-specific, exactly as the distinct individual atoms would be in a crystal (Kozloski et al., 2001). Presynaptic layer 5 neurons were excited to fire by laser-induced, localized uncaging of glutamate. After bulk loading of many neurons with the calcium indicator Fura AM, the cells postsynaptic to the excited presynaptic cell were identified using calcium imaging. Three stereotyped classes of postsynaptic follower cells were identified: large triangular interneuron, fusiform interneuron, and "dangling" pyramidal neuron. Astonishingly, the relative positions of the somata of the presynaptic neuron and the follower cells were found to be ordered and nonrandom. For example, the large triangular interneuron tended to be positioned above the presynaptic cell, whereas the fusiform interneuron was offset horizontally, with the dangling pyramidal cell positioned below the presynaptic cell (Fig. 3.5). The apparent existence of such ordered, subtype-specific, crystal-like arrangements in cortical networks for both interneurons and excitatory cells underlies the immense potential of the Cajal-paradigm and suggest that the achievement of the great synthesis may only be a question of time. It is interesting to note here that crystal-like arrangements of cortical neurons may also exist in the functional domain, in the representation of the geometry of the environment, as recent results indicate that neurons in the dorso-caudal entorhinal cortex fire repeatedly when an animal's position

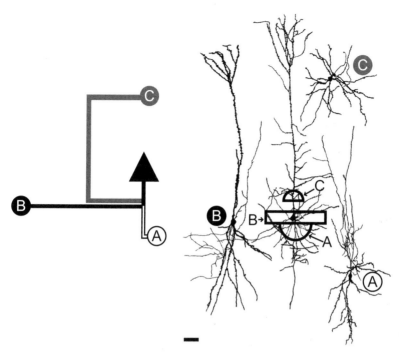

Figure 3.5 **Specificity of layer V subcircuits.** A layer V corticotectal pyramidal "trigger" neuron (second cell from the left; axons and dendrites are both shown) surrounded by examples of three stereotyped classes of postsynaptic "followers" (axons shown with thinner lines) identified by optical probing: large triangular interneuron (cell C), fusiform interneuron (cell A), and "dangling" pyramidal neuron (cell B). Somata of neurons from each class were found in stereotyped regions surrounding the trigger neurons. These regions are depicted as letter-coded shapes surrounding the corticotectal soma. Each shape contained all somata of the corresponding follower class, with the exception of a single pyramidal follower, which was offset medially from the trigger due to a distortion in the cortical plane within this slice. Scale bar, 50 μm. These results from Kozloski et al. (2002) indicate that a circuit diagram (upper left) specifying neuronal classes (shades of gray) and soma positions (circles) will emerge from extensive studies of the cortical microcircuit. Based on the original findings in Kozloski et al. (2001). Adapted, with permission, from Nelson (2002).

coincides with the vertices of a grid of triangles that precisely covers the entire surface of the rat's environment (Hafting et al., 2005; see also Buzsáki, 2005).

4

Cracks in the Crystal: Elusive Neurospecies and the Great Correlation Hunt

----

> *... nature seems unaware of an intellectual need for convenience and unity, and very often takes delight in complication and diversity.*
>
> S. Ramón y Cajal (1906)

Neuronal Species: Can't Live with Them, Can't Live without Them

As detailed in the previous chapter, there is little doubt that interneuronal subtypes or "species" do exist, and that it makes sense to continue to arrange our current knowledge and plan future research concerning interneurons according to subgroups. The concept of interneuronal species is not only central to interneuronal classifications upon which much of our knowledge about interneurons is based, but it is also crucial for determining the fate of interneuronal populations in development and in pathological states. Therefore, it is important to define what we actually mean by interneuronal "subtypes," "subgroups," or "species," three essentially equivalent terms that are used interchangeably by researchers to designate the unit of classification schemes.

The exact definition of a cellular species within an organ in a multicellular organism (in our particular case, interneuronal species in cortical networks) is fraught with challenges. Perhaps as a measure of the difficulties involved, no widely accepted, general definition of interneuronal species exists; in fact, few, if any, have even been suggested. Of course, the concept of species is notoriously difficult to define in precise terms even in the case of animal or plant species. The common definition of animal or plant species involves a group of individuals with the potential for the successful production of fertile offsprings via sexual reproduction. Or, more precisely, here is the widely used species definition by Ernst Mayr (1942): "Species are groups of actually or potentially interbreeding populations, which are reproductively isolated from other such groups." This definition works well in most situations; however, it has its serious limitations. For example, it obviously does not apply to species that reproduce asexually or to individuals beyond the reproductive age. In spite of these problems, biologists continue to heavily rely on the concept of species, in part because the theoretical problems are outweighed by the practical, didactic, and heuristic benefits.

Of course, one can adopt a similarly practical approach to interneuronal species without seeking a formal definition. Nevertheless, it is important to probe and discuss the limitations of the concepts that underlie the idea of interneuronal species. As we alluded to before, interneuronal species definitions primarily involve postsynaptic target specificity and the expression of species-characteristic markers (e.g., parvalbumin, somatostatin, etc.). Although the species definitions based on the postsynaptic targets and on the species-characteristic markers work reasonably well in many situations, they can and do run into problems. For example, the postsynaptic target specificity is rarely absolute. Basket cells often show a strong preference for somata (e.g., 50.6% of the synapses from CA1 basket cells were on pyramidal cell somata in Buhl et al., 1994a), but the postsynaptic targets typically also include proximal dendrites, and, in rarer cases, even axon initial segments as well (Buhl et al., 1994a, 1995). Therefore, although it is straightforward to identify a cell as a basket cell if it has its postsynaptic targets distributed between the soma, proximal dendrites, and axon initial segment in a neat, prototypical 100%:0%:0% or at least in a 90%:10%:0% ratio, the task becomes considerably more difficult and less clear if the target distribution is, say, 40%:55%:5%. This issue is not simply a hypothetical one, as such nontrivial (occasionally labeled as "atypical") target distributions are encountered in practice. For example, the postsynaptic targets of intracellularly recorded and filled hippocampal basket cells mentioned above included proximal dendrites at a rate of around 45% (Buhl et al., 1994a, 1995). Similarly, in vivo intracellularly recorded and horseradish peroxidase-filled cat visual cortical large basket cells and clutch cells (a type of small basket cells) made approximately 20% to 40% of their synapses on somata, the rest on dendrites and spines (Somogyi &

Soltesz, 1986). In other studies, "atypical" hippocampal basket cells
have been described, which innervated somata in about 20% of their
total synaptic targets (Gulyás et al., 1993). Another study defined
"typical" neocortical basket cells as interneurons that (based on light
microscopy) "formed a high fraction (at least 19%) of their putative
synapses on somata of target cells" (Gupta et al., 2000). Bistratified
cells, which are stereotyped as cells specialized to exclusively innervate pyramidal cell dendrites in the strata oriens and radiatum, also
contact somata as well, albeit with a small frequency (4%) (Buhl et
al., 1994a; Halasy et al., 1996). Even in the case of axo-axonic cells,
which are undoubtedly the most stereotyped interneurons, about
10% of the targets were reported in one study to include somata and
proximal dendrites (Buhl et al., 1994a). Note that it has been suggested that the presence of nonstereotypic or "atypical" axo-axonic
cells may be related to the experimental animals being kept in standard laboratory cages representing a deprived environment
(Somogyi & Klausberger, 2005). We will return to this interesting and
important point later in chapter 8.

One solution to these problems could be to agree on some arbi-
trary boundaries for each cell type (e.g., to jointly declare that any
cell with a less than, say, 20% preference for soma is not a basket
cell), but what is perhaps even more important is to realize that when
we categorize (which we undoubtedly need to do for many purposes), we lose information about certain aspects of reality, in
this case, about the preferential, yet often heterogeneous distribution of postsynaptic targets of individual interneurons. A com-
pounding problem is, of course, if the investigator does not perform
the painstakingly labor-intensive, EM-level investigation for each cell
to determine the actual distribution of postsynaptic targets. In such
cases (i.e., when the morphological analysis of biocytin-filled
interneurons is done exclusively and nonquantitatively at the light
microscopical level), all one can use as a point of reference is layer-
specificity. Consequently, it becomes even harder to distinguish
between, say, a bona fide basket cell, an axo-axonic cell, and a trilaminar cell.

In addition to the problems concerning the analysis of the postsynaptic target distribution and interneuronal species definitions,
there are frequently serious challenges with the identification of
markers present in interneurons as well. For example, the lack of
immunoreactivity does not constitute a proof for the true lack

of expression for the peptide in question, and whole cell patch clamp recordings frequently result in an apparent weakening of the immunreactivity (perhaps due to washout of intracellular ingradients from the recorded interneurons). Of course, all of these problems related to interneuronal identifications are multiplied when development or pathological states are studied. As briefly mentioned in chapter 2, several key interneuronal markers are simply not expressed before birth (in rodents), and some (e.g. parvalbumin) start to get expressed only toward the end of the first postnatal week. Regarding neurological disorders, interneurons can change their dendritic and axonal morphologies in diseased states (Davenport et al., 1990; Deller et al., 1995; Mathern et al., 1997; Wittner et al., 2001, 2002), including the possibility of cross-layer axon sprouting, which can confound straightforward classifications. Furthermore, the species-defining marker can be downregulated in an activity-dependent manner in pathological states (Wittner et al,. 2001), adding a whole new level of difficulty to the already complex issue of interneuronal identification.

Getting Lost in Parameter Space: The Mirage of Blind Phenotypic Correlations

Interneuronal researchers obviously cannot use Mayr's deceptively simple criteria (Mayr, 1942; see above) for animal and plant species for defining interneuronal species. Thus, the identification of interneuronal groupings has traditionally relied on the existence of phenotypic markers, such as the postsynaptic target specificity discussed above and the presence or absence of certain marker proteins. Given the fact that there can be a virtually (or, at least, practically) unlimited number of phenotypic markers, the question arises whether it makes sense to blindly "pile up" phenotypic markers and hope that the cellular species would somehow automatically emerge. We could represent the essence of this automatic, blind, or unsupervised approach the following way. Let's consider postsynaptic target specificity first, and plot the percent of somatic synapses made by a given interneuron on the x_1 axis. As discussed above, most cells commonly considered basket cells would fall somewhere between about 20% and 60% on this axis, the axo-axonic cells would be somewhere between 0% and 10%, whereas some other cell types (e.g., bistratified cells and OLM cells) would cluster close to zero. Because in this imaginary example we have two clear clusters, the basket cell cluster and the second cluster containing the obviously mixed group of axo-axonic, bilaminar, and the OLM cells, it would make sense to add a second dimension (e.g., the % of synapses made on initial segments) and plot that on the x_2 axis. On the plane formed by the x_1 and the x_2 axes, therefore, we would have now three clusters, the basket cell cluster, the axo-axonic cluster, and the less heterogeneous but still mixed cluster made up of the bilaminar and OLM cells. We could then add a third axis, x_3, which could represent the percent of the synapses given by the interneuron in question to the proximal dendrites (we could define "proximal dendrites" more precisely, e.g., the dendritic segment between the soma and the first branch-point on the dendrite, or in some other way), resulting in a separation of the bilaminar cells (which give a large percent of their synapses to the proximal dendrites) from the OLM cells (which innervate the distal dendrites).

The hope is, of course, that the cluster of points formed by the various groups in this three-dimensional space would be non-overlapping, even after adding the other cell types that are defined by their unique postsynaptic target specificity, especially the trilaminar cells. Naturally, the goal is to find distinct clusters that could be considered to be separate species. However, it is clear that postsynaptic target specificity alone cannot separate all the separate groups that evidently exist (see Fig. 3.1). Therefore, we need to add more axes to our parameter space, for example, one that would define the location of the cell body in a particular layer in a yes or no fashion (e.g., cell body in the alveus-oriens layer = 1, otherwise 0; note that we use the somatic location here to illustrate the "blind" classification approach; however, in practice, the location of the soma in terms of layers is not a good predictor of the interneuronal subtype). Because there are at least five major CA1 layers, we would have to add at least five additional axes, resulting in a total of eight axes. We could, however, reduce the number of axes by certain tricks; for example, we could plot the distance of the cell body from the bottom of the alveus to the top of the lacunosum-moleculare layer on a single axis (instead of adding separate axes for each of the major layers), in which case we would need only a minimum of four axes.

In a sense, the definition of an interneuronal "species" is the existence of coordinate ranges on these four (or however many) axes that delineate and contain a distinct, well-separated cluster of cells. In principle, any cell could be plotted on this imaginary four-dimensional plot to determine if it is within or outside of, say, the basket cell cluster. Of course, the hope is that the cluster formed by, for example, the basket cells would show zero overlap with the cloud formed by any other cell types. One could also imagine that progress in the field of interneuronal research could be represented by the addition of new, separate clouds (discovery of completely new species) or by the splitting of existing clouds (discovery of separate species within a previously unified group).

However, the main problem with this particular approach is that the number of axes tends to grow, either because the dendritic layer-specificity need to be also considered for species definitions (note that, in the above example, we only considered the axonal target specificity and the location of the soma), or new axes are added as a result of new markers being discovered. In some celebrated cases, the discovery of new markers matches perfectly with existing markers, either showing near-perfect coexpression or near-exclusive complementarity. For example, basket cells (defined based on post-synaptic target preference), as discussed in the previous chapter, express either parvalbumin or CCK, but never both, and PV^+ and CCK^+ basket cells have clearly distinct molecular (e.g., CB1 receptors) and anatomical (e.g., excitatory input density) properties. In many cases, however, a new marker does not coalign perfectly with existing clusters (defined on the basis of postsynaptic targets speci-ficity, cell body location, and dendritic patterns). In such cases, therefore, adding the new axis for the novel marker results in a split-ting of the initially well-defined cluster into two separate species, but the only thing that separates the two species is the presence or absence of a single marker, whose functional relevance may not even be known. The goal of interneuronal research then often becomes the finding of additional properties (e.g., projection to the medial septum) that do coalign with the split group, further justifying the separation of a new species. However, it is certainly daunting that there are thousands of proteins expressed in the brain, and any one of these may or may not be expressed in a cell type specific manner. For example, cytoskeletal proteins (belonging to either the neurofil-ament, microtubule, or microfilament families) had not been tradi-tionally studied by interneuronal researchers before the year 2000, and, as a result, they were not taken into account during classifications, in spite of the fact that it is likely that the axonal, somatic, and dendritic structure and shape of interneurons are strongly influenced, and perhaps even determined, by cytoskeletal proteins. Recent studies, initially conducted for different reasons (specifically, to examine molecular correlates of the reported differences between the mechanical stability of distinct cell types in the dentate gyrus; Toth et al., 1997a), found a stunningly different interneuronal distribution pattern for virtually every cytoskeletal protein that was examined (Ratzliff et al., 2000, 2001). Some cytoskeletal proteins correlated and coaligned perfectly with known markers of distinct interneuronal types (e.g., neurofilament heavy with parvalbumin), and others were apparently coexpressed with a seemingly heterogeneous group of cells (e.g., alpha-actinin). Considering that there are at least 100 different cytoskeletal proteins known, with many more likely to be discovered, the possibility that each of these proteins may have the potential to split the existing interneuronal classes into further subgroups is certainly a reason to pause and reflect on the widely employed, albeit often only implicit, conceptual framework employed by interneuronal researchers. In fact, as we shall discuss in detail later in chapter 7, there are now concrete examples where the the inclusion of a set of criteria (similar to the addition of extra parameters in the above discussion) can actually reduce the discriminative properties of the other parameters during unsupervised or "blind" clustering procedures applied to interneurons (Cauli et al., 2000).

Imperfect Correlations: Experimenter's Errors or Reality?

The above-described approach is thus a primarily correlation-based approach (i.e., it is based on the existence of clear correlations among the various, experimentally determined parameters) that rests on the assumption that interneurons fall into distinct clusters and that they do so in a relatively low-dimensional parameter space, certainly before the number of axes becomes high enough to be in the same order of magnitude as the total number of GABA cells in a given brain area. In the latter case, of course, every interneuron would be a separate species, defeating the whole point of classification (as we shall see below, this latter scenario was raised in a recent study). In fact, primarily anatomical investigations, when morphological and immunocytochemical parameters are studied and correlated, tend to show, for the most part, the existence of distinct interneuronal subgroups, generally supporting the idea that interneuronal species indeed do exist, and that these subgroups constitute useful grounds for further research. However, the reality experienced by many interneuronal researchers who attempted to correlate physiology (typically, based on examination of sustained depolarizing current pulse-evoked firing properties in vitro, or, in rarer cases, the response to neuromodulators) with axonal and dendritic anatomy (with or without immunocytochemistry for additional markers) frequently seemed to contradict, or at least weaken, the contention that interneurons fall into neat categories, especially when only a few defining parameters could be studied simultaneously for each recorded cell.

As an example, Table 4.1 shows intracellularly recorded CA1 interneurons that were found to be immunoreactive for CCK from a recent study (Pawelzik et al., 2002). As is evident from the list, CCK-positive interneurons could be found in many layers, their dendrites were oriented in several directions and extended to various distances, but all these tended to coalign with the axonal arbor. Considerable heterogeneity emerged, however, when a physiological parameter was considered as well (i.e., the pattern of cell discharges). For example, even if we focus on an anatomically homogenous-looking group such as the CCK$^+$ cells with somatic locations in the stratum pyramidale and uniformly vertical soma-dendritic orientation, with dendrites extending from the alveus to the stratum lacunosum-moleculare, and axonal arbors that are basket-like, the cell discharge patterns still turned out to be highly heterogeneous, from regular spiking (three cells) to fast spiking (one cell) and burst firing (two cells).

Because correlating the physiological properties of cells to anatomically defined interneuronal subclasses was rightly judged to be crucially important for further progress, many laboratories have been involved in a "correlation hunt," starting with the mid-1980s and continuing up till today. In spite of this effort, there have been a stream of studies reporting only partial and imperfect correlations, similar to those described above in connection with Table 4.1, between the anatomically defined interneuronal cell types and physiological properties such as discharge characteristics (Lacaille & Schwartzkroin, 1988; Spruston et al., 1997; Ali et al., 1999; Gupta et al., 2000) or the response to neuromodulators (Parra et al., 1998;

Table 4.1   Properties of parvalbumin-immunoreactive (PV-IR) and colecystokinin-immunoreactive (CCK-IR) interneurons.

Chemical marker	Somatic location	Soma-dendritic orientation	Dendritic extent	Axonal arbour	Cell discharge	No.
PV+	SP	Vertical	Alv-SLM	Basket	FS	18
PV+	SP	Vertical	SO-SLM	Basket	FS	2
PV+	SO	Vertical	Alv-SLM	Basket	FS	3
PV+	SO	Vertical	Alv-SR	Basket	FS	1
PV+	SR	Vertical	Alv-SLM	Basket	FS	1
PV+	SP	Vertical	Alv-SLM	Basket	RS	1
PV+	SP	Vertical	Alv-SLM	Basket	BF	3
PV+	SP	Vertical	SO-SR	Bistratified	FS	3
PV+	SP	Vertical	Alv-SR	Bistratified	FS	1
PV+	SP	Vertical	Alv-SLM	Bistratified	RS	1
PV+	SO	Vertical	Alv-SLM	Bistratified	FS	1
PV+	SR	Vertical	Alv-SLM	Axo-axonic	FS	1
CCK+	SP	Vertical	Alv-SLM	Basket	RS	3
CCK+	SP	Vertical	Alv-SLM	Basket	FS	1
CCK+	SP	Vertical	Alv-SLM	Basket	BF	2
CCK+	SO	Vertical	Alv-SLM	Basket	FS	2
CCK+	SO	Horizontal	Alv-SO	Basket	RS	1
CCK+	SR	Vertical	Alv-SR	Basket	RS	1
CCK+	SR	Vertical	Alv-SLM	Basket	RS	1
CCK+	SR/ SLM	Vertical	SO-SLM	Basket	RS	1
CCK+	SR/ SLM	Vertical	Alv-SLM	Basket	RS	1
CCK+	SR	Vertical	Alv-SLM	Trilaminar	RS	1
CCK+	SP	Vertical	Alv-SLM	Bistratified	FS	1
CCK+	SP	Vertical	Alv-SR	Bistratified	RS	1
CCK+	SP	Vertical	Alv-SR	Bistratified	FS	1
CCK+	SO	Vertical	Alv-SLM	Bistratified	RS	1
CCK+	SO	Horizontal	Alv-SO	SO-SO cell	FS	1
CCK+	SR/ SLM	Horizontal	Alv-SLM	Quadrilaminar	RS	2
CCK+	SR/ SLM	Horizontal	SR-SLM	Schaffer-associated	RS	4
CCK+	SR/ SLM	Horizontal	SO-SLM	Schaffer-associated	FS	1
CCK+	SR/ SLM	Horizontal	SR-SLM	Perforant path–associated	BF	1

Alv, alveus; BF, burst-firing; FS, fast-spiking; RS, regular-spiking; SLM, stratum lacunosum-moleculare; SO, stratum oriens; SP, stratum pyramidale; SR, stratum radiatum.
Reprinted, with permission, from Pawelzik et al. (2002).

McQuiston & Madison, 1999) (note that, in many cases, papers tend to emphasize the existence of correlations, perhaps because positive findings are more appealing to reviewers and readers alike, even if the actual data frequently reveal the presence of considerable, unexplained heterogeneity as well).

How can we explain the apparently persistent presence of high intragroup variability? Perhaps the most pressing question is whether the intragroup variability is real or due to experimenter error. One possibility is that the apparent intragroup variability arises from the existence of more than a single interneuronal species within the studied population of cells. Indeed, as discussed above in connection with Fig. 3.1, CCK$^+$ basket cells may contain two subgroups (Somogyi & Klausberger, 2005). The other possibility is related to the fact that one can bring up, virtually for all studies, a series of technical issues that may or may not have influenced the strength of the apparent correlations, such as the lack of electron microscopical verifications of the anatomical identity of the intracellularly recorded and visualized cells, the usage of slices as opposed to in vivo recordings, the employment of the unphysiological, prolonged depolarizing current pulses to evoke firing, the exogenous application of neurotransmitter agonists for extended periods of time, sometimes even in a repeated fashion, and many others. However, the high number of studies that failed to find outright, clear-cut correlations between the various studied parameters should make us at least wonder if all these negative findings can be purely ascribed to experimenter errors. If it is not, or not exclusively, experimenter error that we are dealing with here, then why is it so difficult to find these correlations?

One suggestion, aimed at finding a way out of the difficulties posed by the heterogeneity found in these correlated anatomical and physiological studies, was to use more and more parameter axes for correlations. In essence, the argument was that the problem lies with the fact that only too few parameters are used for correlations, and that one needs to find the right combinations of parameters to delineate subgroups. For example, a recent paper (Gupta et al., 2000) suggested that, although there were no correlations between the anatomically defined class (based on light microscopy) and the firing characteristics (evoked by sustained current pulses), distinct groupings could be found when a third parameter, the facilitating or depressing nature of the short-term plasticity properties of the postsynaptic responses, were also taken into account (Table 4.2). Just as most studies that failed to find correlations could be criticized on technical grounds, the latter study that did show correlations also exhibited certain weaknesses that decreased confidence in the conclusions, including the classifications of cells into subgroups based on light microscopy alone without additional immunocyto-chemical markers and the low number of cells that were found in several of the categories (Table 4.2) that raised the question of whether pure combinatorial chance, similar to pulling colored balls from a basket, may have produced at least some of these apparent correlations.

It is interesting to note that most reports of strong, reliable cor-relations between the parameter axes came from structural or immunocytochemical studies (Freund & Buzsáki, 1996), but much fewer from combined morphological and in vitro physiological approaches where firing patterns were considered in response to square depolarizing current pulses. In fact, as we shall see in subse-quent chapters, there may be perfectly legitimate reasons why it was especially the attempts at correlating firing patterns with anatomical cell classes that frequently ran into difficulties. Furthermore, as we shall argue later in chapter 8, there may be important physiological reasons why considerable cell-to-cell variability exists in major func-tionally relevant parameters within interneuronal populations.

Table 4.2   Summary of GABAergic innervation of pyramidal cells.[a]

Anatomy	Physiology	Synapse	Number of cases
Mapping synaptic classes onto neuronal anatomy			
BC		F2	12
SBC		F1	3
		F2	3
		F3	3
NBC		F2	12
		F3	5
MC		F2	11
		F3	2
BTC		F2	10

(Continued on the following page)

Anatomy	Physiology	Synapse	Number of cases
	Mapping synaptic classes onto neuronal physiology		
	c-AC; b-AC	F1	7; 2
	c-AC; d-AC; b-AC	F2	20; 4; 1
	c-NAC; d-NAC	F2	16; 23
	c-NAC; d-NAC; b-NAC	F3	4; 2; 1
	b-STUT	F1	2
	c-STUT	F2	4
	c-STUT; b-STUT	F3	4; 2
	Mapping synaptic classes onto combined neuronal anatomy and physiology		
BC	c-NAC	F2	6
	d-NAC	F2	3
SBC	c-AC	F1	3
	c-NAC	F3	3
	d-NAC	F2	2
NBC	c-AC	F2	4
	b-STUT	F3	1
	d-NAC	F2	6
	c-NAC	F3	1
MC	c-AC	F2	3
	b-STUT	F3	1
	c-NAC	F2	4
BTC	c-AC	F2	2
	d-NAC	F2	2

[a]Mapping of GABAergic synapses (F1 to F3) according to presynaptic interneurons defined with anatomical (first section), electrophysiological (second section), and a combination of both anatomical and electrophysiological criteria (third section). Synaptic classification is according to facilitated (F1), depressed (F2), and recovered (F3) recovery test response (RTR) (examined by eliciting short trains of precisely timed action potentials in interneurons across a range of discharge frequencies from 5 to 70 Hz, followed by a RTR 500 ms later; the RTRs were either facilitated, depressed, or unchanged as compared with the first response in the action potential train, suggesting that GABAergic synapses differ in the extent to which they undergo synaptic depression and facilitation). Anatomical classes: Basket cells (BCs); nest basket cells (NBCs); small basket cells (SBCs); Martinotti cells (MCs); bitufted cells (BTCs). The electrophysiological responses presented as three main classes and eight distinct subclasses. The authors proposed a broad classification into nonaccommodating (NAC), accommodating (AC), and stuttering cells (STUT). These major classes were further subdivided into three subclasses according to (i) the presence of a burst response at the onset of the step depolarization (b-NAC, b-AC, b-STUT), (ii) a delay of variable duration until the onset of AP discharge (d-NAC, d-AC), and (iii) the absence of either a burst or a delay in the response, referred to as a classical response (c-NAC, c-AC, c-STUT).
Reprinted, with permission, from Gupta et al. (2000).

It should also be recognized that correlations or classifications based on firing properties tend to run into difficulties for another reason, as argued eloquently in a recent article by Mircea Steriade (2004). The four major types of neocortical neurons distinquished on the basis of firing patterns are the regular-spiking cells (exhibiting single spikes that show adaptation; most pyramidal cells belong to this category), the intrinsically bursting cells (firing clusters of axtion potentials with spike inactivation followed by hyperpolarization and silence), the fast-rhythmic-bursting neurons (giving rise to high-frequency spike bursts in the range of 300 Hz to 600 Hz, which can recur at fast rates, around 30 Hz to 50 Hz), and the fast spiking neurons (generating fast action potentials in a sustained manner without frequency adaptation; e.g., the PV^+ basket cells belong to this category) (Connors & Gutnick, 1990; Gray & McCormick, 1996; Steriade et al., 1996, 1998). Although these categories are widely used and are helpful, in vivo in freely moving animals even slight changes in membrane potentials during shifts in vigilance can transform some of these types into another, even within the same neuron (Steriade, 2004). Thus, the firing patterns of the four major neocortical cell types are not inflexible entities; in fact, variations in firing patterns may play important roles in the participation of different neuronal groups in various oscillatory behaviors across the waking-sleep cycle.

The Other Extreme: Each Interneuron as an Unclassifiable Individual

In a direct challenge to the status quo in interneuronal research, a somewhat tongue-in-cheek, but highly thought-provoking and innovative study took the approach of piling up more and more parameter axes literary, and arrived at some troubling conclusions (Parra et al., 1998). Specifically, Parra and colleagues recorded from a large number of CA1 hippocampal interneurons in slices and measured a number of physiological parameters, including details of firing properties and the responses to various neurotransmitters and neuromodulators, specifically, metabotropic glutamate receptor agonists, serotonin, noradrenaline, and muscarinic cholinergic agents. The essence of the classification relied on the layer-specificity of the axonal arbor, the position of the soma, the layer-specificity of

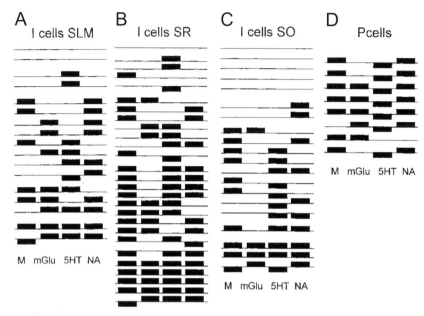

Figure 4.1   **Heterogeneity of interneuron expression of receptors for four modulating transmitters (A–D).** Inhibitory and pyramidal cell responses to neurotransmitter agonists are represented as a bar code with each horizontal line corresponding to a different cell. A bar above the line represents an excitation, a bar below the line an inhibition, and no bar indicates no effect. Tests were made at holding potentials between -60 and -55 mV, and a change in membrane potential of more than 5 mV was counted as an effect. Interneurons (I cells) are separated according to location in stratum lacunosum-moleculare (SLM; n = 17), stratum radiatum (SR; n = 27), and stratum oriens (SO; n = 20). Responses of eight CA1 pyramidal cells (P cells) to the same neurotransmitters are also shown under P cells. Although pyramidal cell responses to these transmitter agonists were rather constant, 25 distinct combinations of responses were detected from the 63 interneurons tested. Reprinted, with permission, from Parra et al. (1998).

the dendrites, and the goal was to determine if cells defined based on these morphological criteria coalign with firing properties, the presence or absence of inward rectification in response to hyperpolarizing current pulses, and with the depolarizing or hyperpolarizing or lack of effect of the bath-applied neurotransmitter receptor ligands. Surprisingly, virtually none of the anatomically defined cells appeared to correlate well with any of the physiological criteria (Fig. 4.1). In fact, if one takes the results literary and pushes the interpretations to the extreme, the inescapable conclusion put forward, only half in jest, by the authors was to declare each interneuron its own kind. In a sense, the implication of the study was that, by examining more and more parameter axes, we are likely to keep splitting the interneuronal groups, and, as the possible number of anatomical, physiological, and biochemical–molecular properties that can be simultaneously examined, at least in principle, is extremely high, we can end up with a situation where each interneuronal "group" contains only a single individual cell. Of course, again, one can come up with a number of critical points regarding this study (e.g., consecutive applications of different second messenger–dependent receptor ligands are difficult to interpret, as the effects of the drugs are virtually impossible to completely reverse upon washout within a short period of time). However, the chief importance of the study lies in the fact that it highlighted the conceptual and technical difficulties in trying to classify interneuron groups by examining an enormously high number of different anatomical, physiological, and pharmacological parameters. As pointed out by the authors, an alternative explanation of their results is that there are interneuronal subgroups, but their number is much higher than we previously imagined. We will return to this latter point in chapter 8, when we address the question of the upper limit in the number of interneuronal species.

5

Functions of Heterogeneity: Meaning of Means and Variability of Variances

---

No one supposes that all individuals of the same species are cast in the same actual mould.

Charles Darwin (1859)

Reconciling Order and Variability: Distinct Subtypes and Cell-to-Cell Heterogeneity as Simultaneously Existing Reality

In the previous two chapters, we have outlined two seemingly contradictory sets of results. On the one hand, chapter 3 highlighted the abundance of evidence indicating that distinct interneuronal subtypes exist, and that the basic differences in axo-dendritic morphology and key marker substances are reliable predictors of functionally important properties. On the other hand, chapter 4 showed that there was also evidence for considerable variability in interneuronal populations, even if one focuses on seemingly homogenous subtypes. Which of these two sets of findings reflects reality? Is it order or variability that dominates the world of interneurons?

Starting with this chapter, in the rest of the book we hope to convince the reader that order and variability are simultaneously existing, equally important facets of cortical networks. But beyond that, we will also put forward the key argument that both order and variability have their own, separate functional roles in the normal and abnormal behaviors of neuronal networks. In fact, we will also contend that the distinction between order and variability is artificial, as there are indications that the degree of variability in various interneuronal parameters is itself ordered and not just present by chance and that it is likely to be closely regulated during development as well as in the adult.

As metioned already in chapter 2, the duality of order and variability holds its origins in the particularities of interneuronal development. Distinct interneuronal populations arise from physically distinct parts of the embryonic forebrain, indicating that differences in interneuronal subtypes have their roots in ontogeny. However, the process of migration of interneurons from their place of birth to their final position in the cortical network is not instantaneous, and interneurons belonging to the very same subtype do not travel in a single, spatially tightly defined cluster. On the contrary, the distance covered by migrating cells is large, and the process of migration is long, and thus it seems likely that interneurons from the same birthplace go through their migratory process with at least some measure of spatial and temporal heterogeneity, even if one considers only a single interneuronal species. Because interneurons continue to receive various, developmentally important signals during the process of migration, the spatial and temporal dispersion must introduce a degree of cell-to-cell variability in distinct interneuronal populations. Added to the developmental origin of order and variability is the naturally occurring local differences in incoming signals and activity levels (e.g., two basket cells in two different parts of the dentate gyrus likely receive nonidentical excitatory and inhibitory inputs and subcortical modulatory influences), which presumably results in further increases in heterogeneity. The point is, therefore, that order and variability in interneuronal populations are not only observed to exist together, but, in fact, this coexistence could not even be otherwise, simply based on what we know about interneuronal development and activity-dependent plasticity processes.

Definitions: Heterogeneity, Variance, and Diversity

In order to elaborate on these thoughts further, we need to first increase the precision of the terms that we use in discussions about interneurons. Most often, the terms "heterogeneity," "variability," and "diversity" are used interchangeably. However, as we shall see in this and in the subsequent chapters, it makes sense to separate these in the following manner (see also Fig. 5.1):

1. **Heterogeneity**: "Interneuronal heterogeneity" is used in the rest of the book as a broad term, referring to either (or both) variability and diversity.

2. **Variability**: The term "variability" is applied here in connection with the variance of a particular parameter. Parameter variance could be derived from any quantitatively measured property, for example, the cell-to-cell variance of the peak sodium current within a population, or the event to event variance in the kinetics of IPSCs, or the synapse to synapse variance of the length of the postsynaptic density, and so forth.

3. **Diversity**: The term "diversity" refers to heterogeneity reflected in the number of subgroups within a population. The term "population" here can refer to either synaptic events or cells. Thus, one can talk about diversity of synaptic events (e.g., inhibitory conductance or G_{IPSC} values that can occur, or the number of clusters/bins in a G_{IPSC} distribution), or the number of cellular categories (interneuronal species). Note that quantitative assessment of diversity includes more than a simple category count, as the relative abundance of the individual categories must also be taken into account (see chapter 6). Note also that we will differentiate between different kinds of diversity (alpha, beta and gamma diversity) in chapter 7.

These definitions are important, because they allow us to be precise about what aspects of interneuronal heterogeneity we want to study or discuss. For example, the term "diversity" should not be used (if one accepts these definitions, that is) to describe the cell-to-cell differences in measurements in some parameter (anatomical or physiological) within a well-defined interneuronal population. Thus, interneuronal diversity may be large (because there are a large number of definable and separable interneuronal subpopulations), with small variability (because the intragroup, cell-to-cell variance is small) in a parameter. Or the situation could be exactly the reverse, where we see small diversity in terms of species numbers but large cell-to-cell variance within the groups. As we shall see later, keeping to these definitions will also allow us to discuss new ways to quantitatively determine variability and heterogeneity. Putting numbers to these terms, in turn, is crucially important for at least two reasons. First, it allows us to compare how the heterogeneity changes in precise, quantitative terms, for example, during development, or during learning, or during a pathological process. Thus, in the future, we will be able to better differentiate between changes in variability (e.g., increased variance of some parameter within a subtype) from changes in diversity (e.g., loss of particular interneuronal subtypes) during the progression of a neurological disease, such as epilepsy. Second, quantifying these terms will also help us to view cell-to-cell variability and species diversity measures as determining closely related but clearly distinct aspects of interneurons.

In order to further illustrate these concepts, let's consider Fig. 5.1. In most studies about interneurons, irrespective of whether the study focuses on synaptic events (e.g., IPSCs) or cellular parameters (e.g., expression of a particular ion channel, or the preferred firing phase of cells during a population oscillation), almost exclusive attention is given to comparisons of means. This mean-centric approach is crucial during the initial establishment of functionally relevant differences between interneuronal subgroups. However, such emphasis on the average behavior misses the other side of the coin, which is that cells do not behave in exactly the same way, even if they belong to the same interneuronal subtype. Clearly, the difference between cells within a subtype may be small, or it may be relatively large, but it is there, and thus it is important to establish, in each case, for every measured parameter, the degree of cell-to-cell variability. As we shall see later in this chapter, the reason why the precise degree of cell-to-cell variance must be better determined and understood in detail is that there is now evidence, from both theoretical and experimental studies, that the degree of variability can significantly influence how networks behave. Similarly, although most current plasticity studies focus on how means change (e.g., during development, or in neurological disease models) (Fig. 5.1A), alterations may also take place in variability (Fig. 5.1B). As we will see later, changes in interneuronal variability may or may not occur simultaneously with changes in means. We will also discuss methods to statistically determine whether an observed, apparent alteration in variance is significant. Figure 5.1C illustrates hypothetical ways that plasticity processes may modulate diversity, either by changing the number of subgroups within a population of synaptic events or by altering the number (and relative abundance) of cellular subgroups that can be defined. Again, it is important to emphasize that changes in any of these three measures (means, variances, and diversity) can occur without concurrent alterations in the other two. Later in this chapter we will show actual examples of such plasticity processes affecting only variances or diversity.

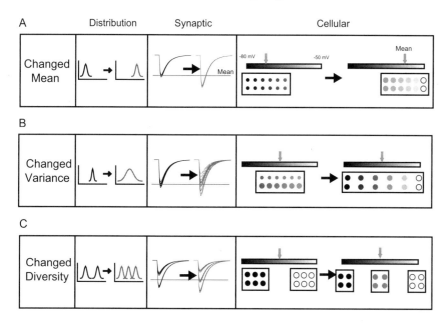

Figure 5.I **Differentiating changes in mean, variance, and diversity.** (A and B) Although most attention is being given to searching for potential alterations in mean values (A) of synaptic and cellular interneuronal properties in various plasticity and neurological disease paradigms, parameters may undergo changes in variance (B), even without alterations in mean values. Changes in a hypothetical distribution of a parameter from control to an altered state are also illustrated. The synaptic parameter is exemplified by the peak IPSC, and the cellular parameter used in the illustration is the resting membrane potential (the circles represent 12 interneurons, shaded according to the resting membrane potential). The mean values are indicated by gray lines in the middle column, and by a vertical downward arrow in the right-hand column. In (A), the population mean changes, whereas the variance change in (B) can occur with or without (as in these examples) a concurrent alteration in the population mean. (C) In principle, diversity of a synaptic or cellular parameter may also change, with or without changes in mean and/or variance. Adapted, with permission, from Santhakumar and Soltesz (2004).

First Look at Variability and Function: Interneuronal Covering of Principal Cells Both in Space and Time

How could we approach the possible functional relevance of cell-to-cell, intragroup variance of certain interneuronal parameters? Figure 5.2 shows a simplified representation of the orderly, spatially segregated innervation of postsynaptic domains along the somato-dendritic axis by distinct classes of interneurons. In an anatomical

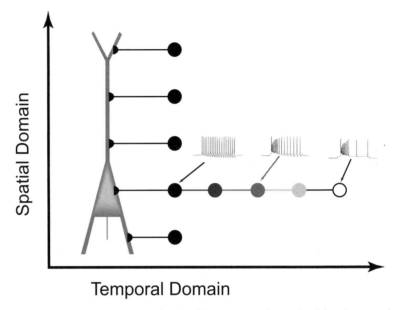

Figure 5.2 **First look at the potential roles of intragroup variance**: Spatial and temporal "covering" of postsynaptic target cells by interneuronal populations. Anatomical segregation of axons according to postsynaptic spatial domains defines major interneuronal species (vertical axis), whereas the intragroup, cell-to-cell variance in action potential accommodation properties within a particular basket cell population is expected to change the dynamic range of interneuronal species.

sense, one may state that the diverse groups of interneurons "cover" the available postsynaptic space, from the initial segment to the distal dendrites. Now let's imagine that each interneuronal subgroup has a certain amount of variability in a functionally relevant parameter, let's say in firing properties. Therefore, within the group of basket cells (for example), we have a certain spread of action potential accommodation rates, from nonadapting through medium adapting to strongly adapting (Fig. 5.2). Because the differential action potential adaptation properties also mean differences in how any given interneuron responds to incoming excitatory signals (e.g., non-adapting cells may be able to better follow inputs coming in at higher frequencies, whereas strongly adapting ones would be expected to be able to respond robustly to slower incoming signals), the degree of variability in firing properties in the basket cell population extends the dynamic range of incoming signals that can activate at least some of the interneurons. Thus, we may say that variability in firing properties means that the given interneuronal population can "cover" the principal cells better in time (note that the loose term "cover" will be made more specific and quantitative later in the chapter; our point here is to introduce the idea). Therefore, in this hypothetical example, we can probably agree that if all basket cells fire in exactly the same way (i.e., if the basket cell population is completely homogenous), there would be certain frequencies of inputs at which the interneurons would not necessarily provide GABAergic inputs to the postsynaptic cell. As the variability increases, the temporal covering of the postsynaptic cell by the interneurons also increases.

Therefore, variability within an interneuronal class may influence the functional behavior of the circuit. If so, we may also hypothesize that perhaps too much variability may also be a problem. For example, if, in a population of interneurons, we start to scatter the cell-to-cell variability in the resting membrane potential, at some point some interneurons may become too hyperpolarized (or too depolarized) to respond to incoming signals altogether. Therefore, we may guess the existence of "optimal" variance for the various parameters. Indeed, if variability is truly important, most biologists would expect that there would be specific mechanisms evolved to regulate it. As we shall see later, although we are far from a complete understanding of the functional relevance and regulation of interneuronal variability, there is now increasing modeling and experimental evidence that support these predictions.

Simulations of Interneuronal Variance and Synchrony

In order to understand in precise, quantitative terms if and how interneuronal variability modulates single cell and network behavior, we need to systematically change various interneuronal parameters and examine its effects. However, there are no currently available experimental techniques that would readily allow us to change cell-to-cell variability in a specific interneuronal population for a functionally relevant parameter without concurrent changes in means. The latter condition is a key point, as we would like to keep the means unchanged so that we can examine the effects of altered variability in isolation, separate from any potentially confounding change in means. Although experimental techniques do not readily lend themselves to this task, computational modeling offers an excellent opportunity to achieve our goal.

Figure 5.3 shows that the placement of differing amounts of Ca^{2+} channels and Ca^{2+}-activated K^+-conductances ($G_{SK,max}$, mimicking SK^+ channels) in model interneurons conferred different action potential properties (Aradi & Soltesz, 2002). Relatively small amounts of N-type Ca^{2+} conductance ($G_{NCa,max}$) and $G_{SK,max}$ resulted in interneurons that responded to a pulse of depolarizing current in a nonadapting manner. In contrast, high levels of $G_{NCa,max}$ and $G_{SK,max}$ led to cells that showed strong action potential adaptation, and medium levels of expression for these channels resulted in adaptation properties in between the two extremes. Therefore, one can change the level of expression of these ion channels in the computer in a population of interneurons in a way that changes only the cell-to-cell variance of the channel expression levels but not the population mean.

Figure 5.4 illustrates what happened when these interneurons were placed in a network consisting of both interneurons and excitatory neurons (Aradi & Soltesz, 2002). The left panel in Fig. 5.4A shows the baseline condition, where the interneuronal population had a small amount of cell-to-cell variance in the $G_{NCa,max}$ and $G_{SK,max}$ expression levels (i.e. the population was fairly homogenous). As demonstrated by several simulation studies (Lytton & Sejnowski, 1991; Golomb & Rinzel, 1993; Wang & Buzsáki, 1996; White et al., 1998; Tiesinga & Jose, 2000; Aradi & Soltesz, 2002), interconnected interneurons that are spontaneously active (e.g., in this case, as a result of a steady depolarizing input, mimicking the ascending muscarinic cholinergic inputs from the medial septum to hippocampal interneurons) frequently synchronize each other through mutual inhibition and settle at a firing rate that is typically close to the "archetypal" gamma frequency (40 Hz). Because the population of interneurons whose activity is shown in Fig. 5.4A (left panel) was fairly homogenous, the interneurons could fire at a high degree of synchrony, in a way that is analogous to a homogenous choir being able to sing in perfect harmony (as all singers are the same). Increasing the cell-to-cell heterogeneity in the interneuronal population, by enhancing the degree of dispersion of the $G_{NCa,max}$ and $G_{SK,max}$ values among the cells resulted in a strongly decreased synchrony in interneuronal firing (Fig. 5.4A, right panel) (Aradi & Soltesz, 2002). Importantly, the increase in variance in the interneuronal parameters (i.e., in the conductance values) was achieved without any alteration in the respective means for these parameters

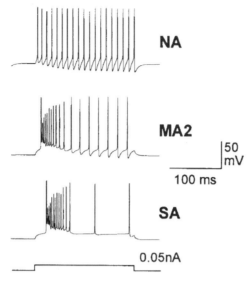

Figure 5.3 **Ion channel expression levels influence firing patterns of model interneurons**: NA, nonadapting; MA2, medium-adapting, type 2; SA, strongly adapting cells. The interneurons possessed five distinct levels of expression for Ca^{2+} and Ca^{2+}-activated K^+ channels (the N-type Ca^{2+} channel conductances ($G_{NCa,max}$) were 7, 11, 13, 17, and 19 mS cm^{-2}, whereas the corresponding SK^+ channel densities ($G_{SK,max}$) were 0.03, 0.07, 0.11, 0.17, and 0.22 mS cm^{-2}). The differing levels of expression for these ion channels conferred different action potential adaptation properties, from nonadapting (NA; for the lowest levels of expression, i.e., $G_{NCa,max} = 7$ and $G_{SK,max} = 0.03$), to medium adapting (MA1, MA2, MA3) and to strongly adapting (SA; with the highest levels of expression) interneurones. All cells started at –60 mV. The current pulse (bottom drawing; 0.05 nA for 200 ms) was delivered from the resting membrane potential. The firing threshold was the same for all cell types. Note that the simulations of distinct expression levels for these two conductances made it possible to create populations of interneurons with various levels of variability (see next figure). Adapted, with permission, from Aradi and Soltesz (2002).

across the population of interneurons. In spite of the fact that the population mean did not change, alteration in interneuronal variability had a clear and strong effect on the functional behavior of the interneuronal network. Again, the choir analogy can help to understand what happened: as the singers became more different from each other, it became harder for them to sing in perfect unison (however, the dynamic range of the ensemble may have increased).

The manipulation of the cell-to-cell variability in these two conductances in interneurons did not affect interneuronal synchronization only. The excitatory ("principal") cells, which were postsynaptic

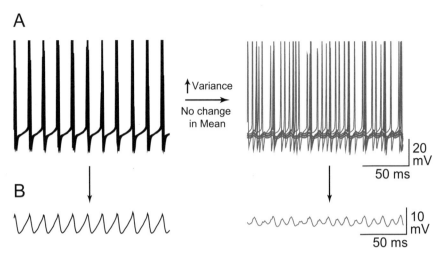

Figure 5.4   **Functional consequences of alterations in parameter variance: Changes in synchrony and subthreshold membrane potential oscillations.** (A) Superimposed traces from 25 model interneurons illustrate that increasing the cell-to-cell variance in Ca^{2+}- and K^+-channel expression (influencing the degree of action potential adaptation) in an interneuronal population decreases the synchrony of gamma frequency (40 Hz) interneuronal firing. (B) Intracellular membrane potential oscillations indicate synchronized IPSPs (left panel) in the principal cells connected to the less heterogeneous interneurons (left panel). As the variance in the interneuronal firing was increased, the IPSPs desynchronized (right panel). Therefore, changes in variance in a single interneuronal parameter, even without changes in means, can influence both interneuronal synchrony and postsynaptic subthreshold oscillations. The original version of this figure appeared in Aradi and Soltesz (2002). Adapted, with permission, from Santhakumar and Soltesz (2004).

to these interneurons, received IPSPs according to the pattern of discharge in the presynaptic interneurons. When the interneurons were homogenous and fired in near-perfect synchrony, the resulting IPSPs were also synchronized and large (Fig. 5.4B, left panel), appearing as intracellularly recorded, large membrane potential oscillations in these model excitatory neurons. As the degree of cell-to-cell variability in the interneuronal population increased and the interneuronal firing became less and less synchronized, these rhythmic IPSPs also became less and less evident (Fig. 5.4B, right panel). Therefore, changes in the variance of interneuronal parameters in a population of interneurons can have robust effects on both the interneurons and on the excitatory neurons. In fact, it has been shown directly (Aradi & Soltesz, 2002) that the excitatory principal cells will respond differently to incoming excitatory inputs, depending on whether they are connected to homogenous or heterogeneous presynaptic interneurons. In the principal cells that received the large, synchronous IPSPs, inhibition was strong for most of the time; however, these cells received virtually no IPSPs just before the quasisynchronous discharges in the interneurons (in a sense, there was a temporary "hole" in the incoming inhibitory inputs). As a result, when EPSPs arrived at this critical point in time, they could discharge the postsynaptic excitatory cells relatively easily. In contrast, the less synchronized IPSPs, arriving from the heterogeneous population of interneurons, were more dispersed in time, resulting in a larger resistance to action potential discharges when the principal cells were challenged with EPSPs (Aradi & Soltesz, 2002). Therefore, interneuronal variability strongly influences how principal cells respond to excitatory inputs. In this particular case, increasing interneuronal variability decreased the excitability of the postsynaptic neurons. Of course, decreased excitability is a good thing if we think of it in terms of preventing runaway seizures, but it is not a good thing if we want the principal cell to fire appropriately (e.g., during coding in hippocampal place cells). Thus, it seems reasonable to assume that the biological network is likely to display a certain, functionally optimal level of interneuronal cell-to-cell variability somewhere between complete homogeneity and maximal heterogeneity. We shall explore this point later.

In the example discussed above, simulations showed that changes in interneuronal cell-to-cell variance can modulate synchrony, intracellular oscillatory patterns, and neuronal excitability. Obviously, there are many possible parameters for which similar variability-effects can be tested. For some parameters, it has been already done; for example, for variance-changes in resting membrane potential and leak conductance, clustering of GABAergic inputs on the postsynaptic site, incoming EPSP phase and frequency (Aradi & Soltesz, 2002). The results indicated that changes in the cell-to-cell variance of a variety of functional and anatomical interneuronal parameters can strongly influence a large number of functionally relevant effects, including modulation of interneuronal and excitatory cell synchrony, firing rates, response to sudden changes in incoming excitation, theta-gamma oscillations, and excitation of postsynaptic cells by interneurons (Aradi & Soltesz, 2002).

Toward Rules that Underlie the Modulation of Postsynaptic Behavior by Interneuronal Variability

Although the previous simulation results determined that, at least in model cells, changes in variability in interneuronal populations can modulate neuronal excitability, the next step is to predict in advance the effects of such alterations in variance. The issue of prediction is especially relevant because, although increased variability in interneurons results in stronger inhibition of postsynaptic cell firing in most cases, there are parameter ranges where increased interneuronal variance decreases inhibition of postsynaptic cells (Aradi & Soltesz, 2002). Therefore, we need to determine if there are rules that underlie the direction and magnitude of the changes in neuronal excitability resulting from altered interneuronal heterogeneity.

In the previous section, we introduced changes in various cellular parameters and looked at their effects on interneurons and postsynaptic principal cells in networks. Although this network-based approach was helpful in determining that variance-effects did indeed exist, it would be useful to simplify our paradigm. Thus, we could take advantage of the fact that all the alterations that occurred in the principal cell behavior after changes in interneuronal cellular parameters (expression of calcium currents) in the previous simulations took place through the GABAergic synapses. For example, changes in interneuronal firing properties modulated the timing of activation of the GABAergic model synapses on the postsynaptic cells. Therefore, in order to better understand how variance regulates neuronal functions, it is sufficient to consider a single postsynaptic cell and its GABAergic synaptic inputs (without the presynaptic interneurons).

Figure 5.5 shows the results of the simulations (Aradi et al., 2002). In panel A, we see that the postsynaptic cell (indicated as a principal cell, or "PC," although the cell could be of any type), in the absence of incoming IPSPs, fired at a certain rate as a result of a constant depolarizing excitatory current input. In B, the upper row shows what happened when the cell received relatively small inhibitory conductances (G_{IPSC}-s) with zero variance (SD = 0). Because the conductance was small, the postsynaptic cell's firing rate decreased somewhat (upper right panel in Fig. 5.5B), compared to panel A (right panel). When the same average (mean) inhibitory conductances were injected into the cell, but now with a certain variability

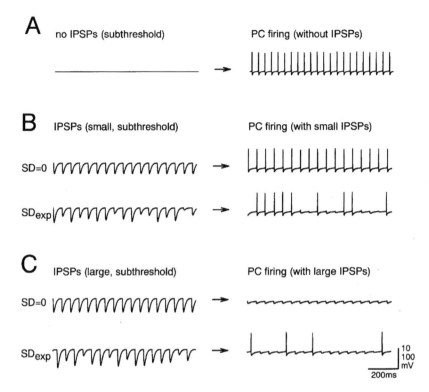

Figure 5.5 **Altered variance in the peak conductance values of IPSC populations significantly changes the efficacy of inhibition.** Note that changes in IPSC heterogeneity were
carried out by alterations in the width (variance), but not the mean, of the IPSC peak
conductance distributions. Left panels: IPSPs (for clarity, the IPSPs are shown with the
cell being kept just below firing threshold); Right panels: Modulation of the firing of the
postsynaptic principal cell (PC) as a result of the IPSPs. (A) The PC firing rate is illustrated when no inhibitory synaptic inputs arrived at the PC. In (B), IPSPs were generated with the same mean IPSC peak conductance, but with either SD = 0 (upper trace)
or with the experimentally measured standard deviation (SD_{exp}) (lower trace). Note the
decreased PC firing with increased heterogeneity in the IPSPs. In this figure, the mean
peak IPSC conductance was equal to 12 times the mean mIPSC conductance = 10.75 nS
(for similar effects around a smaller mean conductance, see Fig. 4 in Aradi et al., 2002),
and the SD_{exp} was 5.51 nS. The IPSC peak conductance values were generated by random draws from Gaussian distributions with the same mean but with either SD = 0 or
with SD_{exp}. (C) Similar to (B), but the mean IPSC conductance was increased (to 16.13
nS, with a concomitant increase in SD_{exp} to 8.26 nS to keep coefficient of variation
unchanged). Note that, with the larger mean IPSC conductance in (C), the PC firing
rate was increased with enhanced heterogeneity of the IPSCs. Reprinted, with permission, from Aradi et al. (2002).

(indicated as SD_{exp}, i.e., the experimentally measured standard deviation of the peak miniature IPSC conductance in the lower left panel in Fig. 5.5B), the firing rate of the postsynaptic cell decreased even more. Therefore, we can conclude from these simple observations that increasing variance can have an effect on the postsynaptic firing rate.

But can we explain the observed effect? The explanation is, in fact, very simple. Because the injected mean conductance was relatively small, the cell continued to fire at a fair rate even in its presence. When we scattered the conductances around the mean, some events were smaller and some larger than the mean (because we introduced the changes in variance without changing the mean conductance). The smaller events made little difference, as the cell was already firing. However, the larger events could cause effective inhibition of spiking (i.e., the largest IPSPs could shut the cell down).

So what would happen if we now increase the mean inhibitory conductance and introduce variability in the synaptic events? As shown in panel C of Fig 5.5, without variance (SD = 0), the larger mean inhibitory conductance could cause complete inhibition of the firing of the postsynaptic cell (note that the cell still received the same amount of depolarizing current input as before). When the events were scattered around this larger mean value (with the SD_{exp} again), the postsynaptic cell's firing rate actually increased (in contrast to what we saw with the smaller mean conductance). Again, the explanation is simple. Because the mean G_{IPSC} was large enough to shut the cell down (upper right trace in Fig. 5.5C), the larger events generated by the increased scatter in the population mattered little (because the cell was already silent). However, when the increased variability produced an event that was small enough, the cell could reach firing threshold and discharge an action potential (Aradi et al., 2002).

From these simple simulation experiments, we can conclude that increases in event-to-event variance in a population of incoming GABAergic events can either decrease or increase postsynaptic cell firing rates, and we can also conclude that the direction of the change depends on the mean value of synaptic events. With small means, increasing variability decreases firing rates (because the larger events matter), however, with large means, increased variability enhances firing rates (because, in this latter case, it is the smaller events that become important).

Figure 5.6 shows the results of the simulation experiments discussed above, with the data plotted in an x–y graph (Aradi et al., 2002). On the x axis, the mean G_{IPSC} is indicated (in units of the experimentally determined mean miniature IPSC conductance) with zero variance (i.e., at each mean, a completely homogenous population of G_{IPSC}-s was injected into the model cell). The y axis shows the cell's firing rate. With no inhibition, the cell fired at around 20 Hz (due to a certain amount of depolarizing current input). As the mean G_{IPSC} was increased, the firing did not change significantly, as long as the mean inhibitory conductance was relatively small (with respect to the depolarizing current input). At a certain point, however, the IPSPs became strong enough to shut the cell down. Let's call the position of this nonlinearity in the plot a "critical point" (or "critical region," depending on how abrupt the drop in firing is with a small increase in the mean G_{IPSC}).

Now we can fully explain and predict the variance-effects observed in connection with Fig. 5.5. If the inhibitory conductance mean is smaller than the critical value, scattering events around that mean (indicated by "B" in panel A in Fig. 5.6) initially has very little effect on the mean firing rates, as long as the degree of scattering is relatively small. As the degree of scattering increases, however, some events will be large enough to reach the critical value and shut the cell down, causing a drop in the average firing rate. These data are shown in Fig. 5.6B. Obviously, the closer point "B" (i.e., the mean value) is to the critical region, the smaller the variance-change needed to produce events that are large enough to reach the critical region. On the other hand, if the mean of the peak inhibitory conductances is larger than the critical value, the opposite will happen. In this case, scattering the incoming synaptic events around the larger mean (point "C" in Fig. 5.6A) will produce events that will be too small to shut the cell down, causing a rise in the average firing rate (Fig. 5.6C), provided that the increase in scatter is large enough and the mean is not too far from the critical region (Aradi et al., 2002).

Thus, we now have certain rules that can predict the variance-effects. Note that these rules are applicable to increasingly realistic scenarios also, for example, to G_{IPSC}-s that are close to the experimentally measured means of mIPSC conductances, to events that arrive at irregular frequencies, and the variance can be introduced not only in peak conductances but in kinetics as well (Fig. 5.7; for

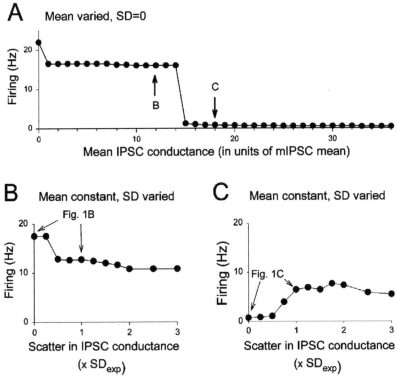

Figure 5.6 **Analysis of the effects of variance in IPSC conductances on firing rates (inhibitory efficacy).** (A) Firing rates of the model PC is plotted against the IPSC conductance (in units of the experimental mean mIPSC conductance = 0.896 nS). Note that, at around 15 times the mean mIPSC conductance (for similar effects at around smaller conductances, see Fig. 4 in Aradi et al., 2002), inhibition became strong enough to shut the cell down, resulting in a region of nonlinearity in the input–output curve. (B) Increasing the variance (from 0 up to $3 \times SD_{exp}$) around the mean IPSC conductance left of the region of nonlinearity in the input–output plot (indicated by the letter "B" in panel A) resulted in a decrease in the PC firing. (C) Increasing the variance around the mean IPSC conductance right of the nonlinearity (indicated by "C" in panel A) decreased PC firing. The depolarizing current injected into the cell to induce tonic firing was $I_{depol} = 0.137$ nA. Reprinted, with permission, from Aradi et al. (2002).

additional details, see Aradi et al., 2002). Furthermore, it is important to realize that the critical region depends on the relative values of excitation and inhibition. For example, increasing the steady excitatory current will shift the critical region to the right (to larger mean τ_{decay} or G_{IPSC} values), as now only longer (or larger) G_{IPSC}s can shut the cell down (Fig. 5.7A). Similarly, changes in the reversal

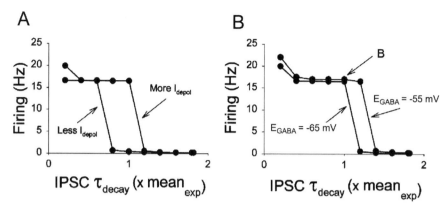

Figure 5.7 **Parameters that determine the position of the region of nonlinearity in the input (IPSC)–output (PC firing) curves.** (A) The position of the region of nonlinearity in the input–output curve was moved to the right or left with more or less depolarizing current (Idepol), that is, it was modified by the strength of the excitation, modeled by the depolarizing current injection. "More I_{depol}" was 0.137 nA, whereas "Less I_{depol}" was 0.136 nA. The IPSC mean conductance was 6.27 nS, with the IPSC mean decay time constant was 6.8 ms. (B) The input–output curve was also modified by changes in the reversal potential for GABA (E_{GABA}). Adapted, with permission, from Aradi et al. (2002).

potential for $GABA_A$ receptor-mediated synaptic currents (E_{GABA}) can also influence the position of the nonlinearity. For example, a depolarizing shift in E_{GABA} will shift the critical region to the right, as only the more prolonged (or larger) mean G_{IPSC}s will be able to inhibit firing (Fig. 5.7B) (Aradi et al., 2002). Thus, in real cells, the critical region will not be a fixed point, but it will likely move around and oscillate on a moment to moment basis, depending on the excitatory inputs arriving at any one point in time and on slight changes in local E_{GABA} values in various points along the somato-dendritic axis. Consequently, scattering events around a certain mean G_{IPSC} input can cause either decreases or increases in firing rates, depending on the state of the postsynaptic neuron.

In summary, the results discussed in this chapter showed that variability in interneuronal parameters, including cellular (e.g., channels influencing interneuronal firing patterns) as well as various synaptic parameters (e.g., peak amplitude and kinetics of the GABAergic conductances), can significantly modulate a number of functional features, including firing rates, oscillatory patterns, and network synchrony (Aradi et al., 2002; Aradi & Soltesz, 2002).

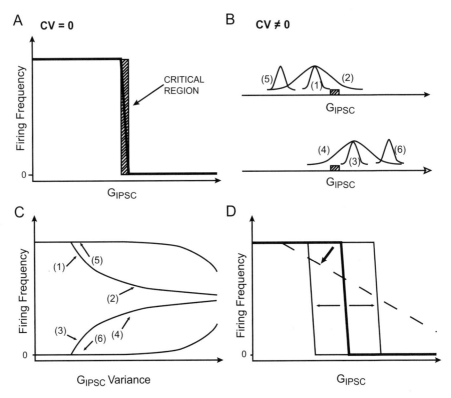

Figure 5.8   **Rules for predicting the effects of changes in input heterogeneity on firing rates.** (A) Schematic drawing of an input–output plot (thick line indicated by "CV = 0"), generated by testing the effects of populations of G_{IPSC}s with CV = 0 on the postsynaptic cell's firing rates (note that the cell fires tonically when G_{IPSC} = 0, as a result of a depolarizing current input). Sharp drop in firing rate (indicated by hatched region) is referred to as the "critical region." (B) Illustration of populations of G_{IPSC}s (Gaussian distributions) used to generate plots in (C). Hatched area indicates location of critical region. (C) When the cell is challenged with populations of G_{IPSC}s that have nonzero CV (indicated by the distributions labeled 1–6 in B), the resulting changes in firing rates can be predicted as indicated by the numbers in (C) (corresponding to the distributions in B). (D) Introduction of stochastic processes (such as irregular interevent intervals) causes a change in the slope of the critical region (dashed line). Changes in tonic depolarization or E_{GABA} causes parallel shifts in the critical region. Reprinted, with permission, from Aradi et al. (2004).

Furthermore, we established some simple rules that allow us to predict the direction of the variance-induced changes, summarized in Fig. 5.8. In the next chapter, we will go beyond these simulations and attempt to enrich these ideas with observations and considerations in real biological neurons.

6

Interneuronal Variability: Plasticity and Regulation

Information is ultimately not derived from species, but from specimens.
Christian Thompson (1997)

Dynamic Clamp-Down on Interneuronal Variance

The simple rules established to test the functional effects of altered variances outlined in the previous chapter were based on observations made in computational model neurons. Clearly, it would be all the more convincing if these interneuronal variance-effects could also be observed in real, biological neurons. As mentioned in the previous chapter, it is currently difficult, if not outright impossible, to systematically change the cell-to-cell variance of a cellular or synaptic parameter in "wet" experiments without confounding changes in means. However, we can use a hybrid system, the dynamic clamp method (Sharp et al., 1993), to achieve our goals, which allows the injection of realistic conductances into neurons with the aid of a computer.

Figure 6.1 shows the effects of injecting realistic, fast GABAergic conductances into biological (i.e., "real") CA1 pyramidal cells. The mean G_{IPSC} is increased along the x axis, and the scatter around each mean is increased from bottom to top along the y axis. The effects of the changes in mean and variances on the cell's firing rates are plotted as a contour plot. Moving up vertically from low to high variances around a high mean ($G_{IPSC} = 17.5$ nS) can powerfully increase the firing rates (as shown in the illustrated example traces in Fig. 6.1). Therefore, alterations in GABAergic input variance can change the firing rates in real biological neurons, even in the absence of changes in mean G_{IPSC} (Aradi et al., 2004), exactly as observed in computational model cells (Aradi et al., 2002). Note also that most

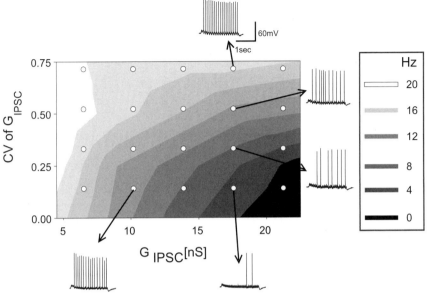

Figure 6.1   **Functional consequences of alterations in parameter variance: Changes in firing rates.** Dynamic clamp results from a hippocampal CA1 pyramidal cell illustrate that the firing rate (gray-scale coded) can be modulated not only by changes in the mean injected GABAergic conductance (G_{IPSC} plotted on the x axis) but also by changes in G_{IPSC} variance (CV = coefficient of variation, plotted on the y axis). Note that moving vertically from low to high variance (e.g., at G_{IPSC} = 17.5 nS) can powerfully modulate the firing rate, even in the absence of changes in mean G_{IPSC}. An original version of this figure appeared in Aradi et al. (2004). Adapted, with permission, from Santhakumar and Soltesz (2004).

of the means plotted in Fig. 6.1 were either within or to the right of the critical region. Therefore, increasing variance resulted in enhanced firing rates, as predicted based by the rules outlined in the previous chapter. Figure 6.2 (Aradi et al., 2004) shows the pericritical region in a biological cell, illustrating that increasing variance left of the critical region decreased firing, whereas the reverse could be observed to the right of the critical region, in full agreement with the predictions based on the simulations in model cells.

As discussed in the previous chapter, the critical region in the model cells could be shifted to the left or to the right by appropriate modifications in the amount of depolarizing current that the cell received (I_{depol}) and by changes in E_{GABA}. The predictions of the modeling studies (Aradi et al., 2002) regarding the effects of I_{depol} and E_{GABA} were also verified in biological CA1 pyramidal cells

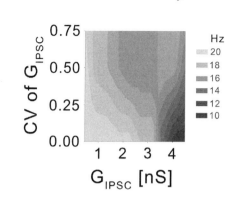

Figure 6.2   **Modulation of firing rates by variance in peak G_{IPSC} in a dynamic clamped CA1 pyramidal cell.** Contour plot for G_{IPSC} means between 0 and 4.5 nS (measured in 10 steps). Note that increasing CV around small mean G_{IPSC}s leads to decreased firing, whereas increasing CV around larger mean G_{IPSC}s results in increased firing. $I_{depol} = 0.9$ nA; $E_{GABA} = -65$ mV; $V_h = -60$ mV. Adapted, with permission, from Aradi et al. (2004).

using dynamic clamp methods. Figure 6.3 illustrates the influence of increasing tonic depolarization on variance-effects around multiple peak conductances. The increase in I_{depol} caused a rightward shift in the contour plots (note the changes in the x-axis in Fig. 6.3), because with the increasing excitation, larger G_{IPSC}s were required to suppress the cell firing (Aradi et al., 2004). In contrast to the rightward shift in the contours with increasing I_{depol}, a hyperpolarizing shift in E_{GABA} caused a leftward shift in the contours (Fig. 6.4), because smaller conductances could suppress the cell firing when E_{GABA} was more hyperpolarized.

Importantly, the rules for the variance-effects apply not only for changes in the scatter in the peak conductances of incoming GABAergic synaptic events, but these rules could be applicable to other parameters as well (Aradi et al., 2004). Figure 6.5 shows the effects of changes in heterogeneity in the decay time constants of GABAergic conductances, with the peak G_{IPSC} amplitude kept at a constant value. As expected, increasing the mean decay time constants (plotted on the x axis in Fig. 6.5) decreased the firing of the cell (at a given I_{depol}). In addition, the scattering of the decay time constants around mean values that were large enough to decrease firing resulted in an increase in the discharge rate of the postsynaptic cell (Fig 6.5), as predicted by the computational simulations (Aradi et al., 2002).

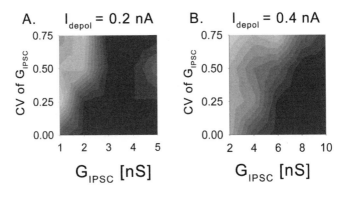

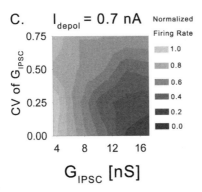

Figure 6.3   **Variance effects change with depolarization.** (A–C) Contour plots illustrating variance effects on firing rates from a dynamic clamped CA1 pyramidal cell at various mean G_{IPSC}s with increasing I_{depol} (E_{GABA} = –65 mV; V_h = –60 mV). Note the changes in x axis range and that the firing rates are normalized for clarity. Adapted, with permission, from Aradi et al. (2004).

Variance-effects were also shown for other parameters, for example, for changes in interevent intervals (Aradi et al., 2004), and they could also be observed in more dynamic settings. For example, how do cells respond to sudden, stepwise changes in G_{IPSC} variance (without concurrent changes in inhibitory conductance means)? Figures 6.6A and 6.6B show that increasing G_{IPSC} variance from the baseline values of CV = 0.25 to 0.5 or to 0.75 in both real and model CA1 cells increased their firing rates, as expected. A slightly different effect could be seen in CA3 cells (Figs. 6.6C and 6.6D). These cells fire in a bursting fashion without incoming GABAergic inputs (see inset; note that a certain amount of depolarizing current was injected into the cells), and the introduction of GABAergic events in both the

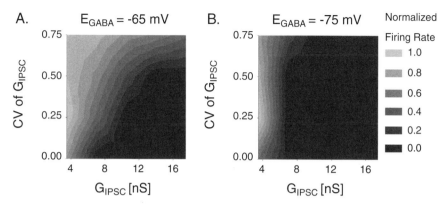

Figure 6.4 **Variance-effects change with alterations in E_{GABA}.** Leftward shift in contour plots from a dynamic clamped CA1 pyramidal cell with a hyperpolarizing change in E_{GABA} (I_{depol} was 0.7 nA; V_h = –60 mV). Adapted, with permission, from Aradi et al. (2004).

real and model cells stopped the rhythmic bursting behavior. Increasing the variance from CV = 0.25 to 0.5 enhanced the firing rates of CA3 cells in a manner similar to CA1 cells. However, stronger sudden increases in CV (to 0.75) resulted in the discharge of a burst in CA3 cells (note that the explanation of this effect is simple: large enough changes in variances in peak G_{IPSC}s will produce sets of small G_{IPSC}s that allow the reappearance of the bursting behavior in CA3 cells) (Aradi et al., 2004). Therefore, we can think of CA3 cells as

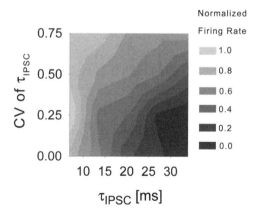

Figure 6.5 **The effects of heterogeneity in G_{IPSC} decay in a dynamic clamped CA1 pyramidal cell.** Figure shows variance effects around various mean G_{IPSC} decay time constants (I_{depol} = 0.7 nA; V_h = –60 mV; E_{GABA} = –75 mV). Adapted, with permission, from Aradi et al. (2004).

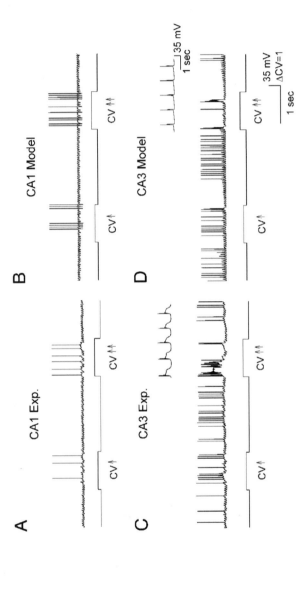

Figure 6.6 **Transient changes in the coefficient of variation of G$_{IPSC}$s in dynamic clamped and modeled CA1 and CA3 pyramidal cells.** (A) Representative trace illustrating changes in firing rates in response to stepwise increases in CV of peak G$_{IPSC}$s (I_{depol} = 0.1 nA; G$_{IPSC}$s: 20 Hz, with a mean value of 7 nS; CV = 0.25 before first step; CV = 0.5 during first step; CV = 0.75 during second step). (B) As in (A), but from a model CA1 cell (I_{depol} = 0.14 nA; G$_{IPSC}$s: 20 Hz with a mean of 2.5 nS). (C) Representative trace illustrating effects on firing rates and firing modes in response to stepwise increases in the CV of peak G$_{IPSC}$s from a CA3 pyramidal cell (I_{depol} = 0.1 nA; G$_{IPSC}$s: 20 Hz with a mean of 10 nS; CV changes as in A). (D) As in (C), but from a simulated CA3 pyramidal cell (I_{depol} = 0.3 nA; mean G$_{IPSC}$ = 12 nS). Note the appearance of burst firing in response to the second step (CV increased to 0.75 from 0.25) in both experimental and simulated CA3 cells (bursts are shorter in model). (C and D, insets) Burst firing alone when the cell receives I_{depol} but not G$_{IPSC}$s. Reprinted, with permission, from Aradi et al. (2004).

being able to detect sudden changes in the heterogeneity of incoming GABAergic inputs and signal the changed variance by a distinct change in firing pattern from single action potential discharges to bursting. In a sense, therefore, CA3 cells may be thought of as a type of "variance-detectors" in the network.

Furthermore, variance-effects could also be observed in both model and real neurons during membrane potential oscillations (Aradi et al., 2004). As shown in Fig. 6.7, augmentation of the peak

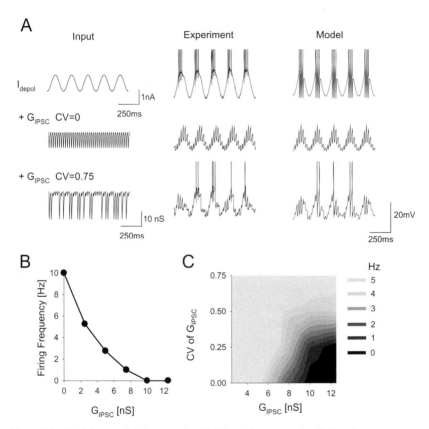

Figure 6.7 **Modulation of firing rates by GABAergic heterogeneity during theta-gamma oscillations.** (A) Representative traces of I_{depol} and G_{IPSC} command inputs (left) and corresponding voltage recordings from a biological (middle) and a model (right) CA1 pyramidal cell (top: $G_{IPSC} = 0$; middle: CV = 0; bottom: CV = 0.75; note that the mean $G_{IPSC} = 12.5$ nS was not changed when CV was increased; $I_{depol} = 5$ Hz sinusoidal current with amplitude oscillating between 0 and 0.5 nA in the experiment and 0 and 0.3 nA in the model). (B) Input–output plot (CV = 0) obtained during theta frequency depolarizations for the biological CA1 cell in (A). (C) Contour plot for the same cell as in (A) and (B). Note that increasing CV enhances firing rates, even if the mean G_{IPSC}s remain unchanged. Reprinted, with permission, from Aradi et al. (2004).

G_{IPSC} amplitude variance (from $CV = 0$ to 0.75, without changes in means) caused dramatic changes in the firing rates of experimental and model CA1 cells during rhythmic intracellular theta-gamma oscillations (the depolarizing current arrived modulated at the theta frequency, whereas the G_{IPSC}s were generated at the faster gamma frequency). Therefore, the behavior of postsynaptic neurons can be modulated by changes in GABAergic synaptic variances in a variety of ways, under many different dynamic conditions, as predicted by the modeling results (Aradi et al., 2002).

Alterations in Variance: Neuromodulators, Neurological Diseases, and Development

The simulation and dynamic clamp results presented on the preceding pages indicate that the degree of cell-to-cell or synaptic event to event variance can have significant functional effects on the postsynaptic cells and on the whole network. Some of the data, especially on variability in cell-to-cell firing properties and interneuronal synchrony, also indicated that the amount of variance is likely to be finely tuned in the neuronal circuits. Too little variance (too much homogeneity) in firing properties generates hypersynchronous interneuronal discharges that lead to large synchronized IPSPs, but it leaves the postsynaptic cell without inhibitory inputs during certain periods (just before the arrival of the synchronous IPSPs) (Aradi & Soltesz, 2002). Too much variance (too much heterogeneity), on the other hand, leads to interneuronal networks that are hard to synchronize (see Fig. 5.4). But what mechanisms may regulate interneuronal variability? This is, in fact, a crucially important question for which there are no solid answers yet.

But there are interesting clues. Although it is not yet clear how population variance of interneuronal parameters is regulated by development, and by normal or pathological forms of activity, any process that differentially affects outliers within a specific population of cells can modulate population variance, at least in principle. For example, slight variations between individual cells in the expression of receptor levels for neuromodulators (e.g., acetylcholine) within an otherwise homogeneous interneuronal population may lead to depolarization of the resting membrane potential after muscarinic activation in some cells but cause only small alteration or no change in others. Such a differential effect of a neuromodulator on a cell population would be expected to lead to an effective increase in the dispersion (variance) of the resting membrane potential values, in addition to a shift in the population mean. Interestingly, muscarinic agonists, similar to several other modulators, have been observed to exert a seemingly puzzling variety of effects on the resting membrane potential of interneuronal populations (Parra et al., 1998; McQuiston & Madison, 1999; Romo-Parra et al., 2003). Although the homogeneity of the studied interneuronal population could have been a potential confounding factor in some of these studies (e.g., biocytin-filled cells that were observed to project to the somatic cell layer in the light microscope could have included both parvalbumin- as well as CCK-positive basket cells, as well as axo-axonic cells), it is likely that a certain, naturally occurring cell-to-cell variance (e.g., in the muscarinic receptor expression level) does exist even in the best-defined interneuronal subpopulation. Such cell-to-cell parameter variance in a cell population could provide the basis for the heterogeneous actions of neurotransmitters and modulators. In fact, based on the astoundingly robust effects of variance-changes in simulation studies, and the likely presence of natural cell-to-cell variance for various neuromodulator receptors among otherwise homogenous interneurons belonging to the same subtype, it has been suggested that regulation of parameter variance in interneuronal populations may be a hitherto unrecognized and possibly key function of subcortical neuromodulatory afferent inputs (Aradi & Soltesz, 2002).

In addition to the short-term alterations in variance that may take place through neuromodulatory processes, there is some evidence that interneuronal intragroup, cell-to-cell variability may undergo long-term alterations in neurological disease paradigms. Figure 6.8A shows the common scenario observed in experimental studies of neurological disease models, where, after a certain manipulation, there is a change in the mean of a certain parameter measured in a number of neurons within a population under scrutiny. Specifically, the data show the resting membrane potential of interneurons located in the granule cell layer in the dentate gyrus from control animals and in animals that underwent moderate fluid percussion head trauma, an experimental model of concussive traumatic brain injury. Note that the resting membrane potential showed a long-lasting depolarizing shift (due to a long-term downregulation of the electrogenic sodium-potassium ATP-ase) after the traumatic impact,

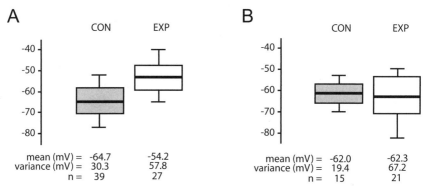

Figure 6.8   **Experimental evidence for altered variance in interneuronal populations in epilepsy.** (A) The resting membrane potentials of interneurons in the granule cell layer of the dentate gyrus show a significant depolarising shift after a single episode of moderate concussive head trauma (Toth et al., 1997a; Ross & Soltesz, 2000). Note that, in this case, only the mean value of the resting membrane potential changed significantly. Con: age-matched, sham-injured controls; Exp: experimental group (after fluid percussion head injury). The analysis of the resting membrane potential was done from samples of 20 seconds as described in Ross and Soltesz (2001). (B) In contrast, the resting membrane potential of interneurones in the stratum oriens of the CA1 region from animals that experienced an episode of experimental prolonged febrile seizures (Exp) (Chen et al., 1999, 2001) did not show any significant alteration in the mean value of the population. However, there was a significant increase in the variance of the resting membrane potential values around the mean across the interneuronal population. In both (A) and (B), box-plots of the data are shown, illustrating the median (horizontal lines close to the middle of the shaded boxes), the 50% of the data around the mean value (shown by the shaded boxes), and the minimum and maximum values (indicated by the vertical "whiskers" sticking out from the boxes). The mean values and the population variance, together with the number of recorded interneurones (n) are shown below the box-plots. Statistical analysis of the data showed a significant ($p < 0.05$) change in the mean in (A) (with a t-test or Kolmogorov–Smirnov test) and a significant change in the variance in (B) (with the variance ratio F-test). Adapted, with permission, from Aradi and Soltesz (2002).

which, as it has been explicitly demonstrated, enhanced the ability of incoming excitatory signals to discharge the interneurons (Ross & Soltesz, 2000, 2001). Note also that, although there was a shift in the mean, there was no obvious change in the variance of the resting membrane potential values between the control and the experimental interneuronal populations. Figure 6.8A shows so-called box-plots of these results (the line in the middle of the box-plots show the median, the box contains 50% of the data points indicating the spread of the data, and the "whiskers" sticking out from the boxes show the maximum and minimum values). Note that the 50% of the interneurons differed from each other by less than 8 mV (represented by the height of the boxes) in both the control and in the posttraumatic groups.

In contrast, interneurons in the stratum oriens layer in CA1 one week after prolonged experimental fever-induced or "febrile" seizures (Chen et al., 1999; this is a model of the most common childhood seizures) displayed the opposite scenario. Here, the interneurons in the control and the experimental groups showed virtually identical means, but there was a large increase in the cell-to-cell variances in the resting membrane potentials measured in the postseizure group (Fig. 6.8B). Specifically, 50% of the interneurons were within 5 mV in control, but this value increased to 12 mV after the febrile seizures (note that there is no cell loss after febrile seizures in this model).

Apart from these data, there are no other currently available reports of experimentally determined changes in interneuronal cell-to-cell variance after some manipulation. However, it is very likely that the lack of reports on variance-changes is at least partly due to the fact that most studies focus on changes in the mean values of experimentally measured parameters. In fact, most commonly used statistical tests (e.g., t-tests) would not indicate any significant alteration if the mean or median does not change, therefore, it is possible that many previously studied, and seemingly unaltered interneuronal parameters did in fact undergo prominent, and possibly functionally significant, modifications in various experimental models of neurological diseases. It is interesting to point out that, although changes may occur both in means and variances, in the example shown in Fig. 6.8B, where a neurological disorder-related alteration in variance of an interneuronal parameter has been observed, the change in variance took place without a change in mean value.

Whether and how cell-to-cell variability may change under other conditions is also not yet well understood. At present, we can only hypothesize that interneuronal population variance may undergo alterations during development, certain naturally occurring plasticity processes and perhaps aging. For example, it is conceivable that during postnatal development, as we alluded to before, there may be differences in the maturational states of individual cells belonging to a certain interneuronal subtype, and, as ontogenetic development progresses toward the adult situation, there is a decrease in the population-level variability. Similarly, cellular heterogeneity may also be exacerbated by aging-related pathological conditions; for example, in Alzheimer's disease in which the progression of pathological change reportedly varies between adjacent neurons (Braak & Braak, 1991), although it is not clear how this observation applies to interneurons specifically. Clearly, future experiments are needed, aimed at determining how interneuronal population variance is altered under various conditions, and the results will give likely provide us with important clues regarding the nature of the underlying regulatory mechanisms as well.

Statistical Methods of Measuring Changes in Variance

A better understanding of variance-changes in interneuronal populations requires somewhat unusual quantitative approaches in terms of statistics. Typically, statistical tests for differences in means or medians have dominated studies into normal and pathological forms of neuroplasticity concerning both principal cells and interneurons, but there is increasing interest in assessing differences in variations that may or may not be associated with differences in means or medians (Santhakumar & Soltesz, 2004; Földy et al., 2005). For example, we may be interested to know not only how a specific group of interneurons (e.g., the CCK-positive basket cells) functions in a particular task *on average*, but we may need to know how typical the average performance is across the cell population. The importance of variations in interneuronal populations was underscored by recent computer simulations (Aradi & Soltesz, 2002) and dynamic clamp experimental studies (Aradi et al., 2004; Földy et al., 2004) discussed above, which showed that alterations in variances in a number of interneuronal and GABAergic synaptic parameters can significantly influence firing rate and synchrony, even in the absence of changes in mean values.

The assumption of normality plays an important role in testing for equality of variances. In the two independent sample situation when we can assume normality (e.g., based on the Kolmogorov–Smirnov normality test), the appropriate statistic to test equality of population variances, irrespective of whether the means are equal, is the variance ratio F-test,

$$F = s_1^2 / s_2^2,$$

where s_1 and s_2 are the standard deviations of the two samples, which has an F distribution under the hypothesis that the population variances are equal (Sprent & Smeeton, 2001).

If we need to compare the variances of two groups without assumptions about normality, the nonparametric Conover squared-rank test can be used (Aradi & Soltesz, 2002; Santhakumar & Soltesz, 2004; Földy et al., 2005). The Conover test for equality of variance is based on the squared ranks of absolute deviations from the means (where the data from both samples is combined before ranking) (Sprent & Smeeton, 2001). Certain statistical packages (e.g., StatXact from Cytel) provide a specific program for the Conover squared-rank test. It should also be noted that when sample sizes are fairly small (which is frequently the case in interneuronal research), the nonparametric test is preferred, as the various normality tests often have trouble with extremely small samples.

Transfer of Interneuronal Variability to Principal Cells: Potential for More Functional States?

Now that we have discussed the evidence indicating that GABAergic cell-to-cell or synaptic event to event variance can have significant functional effects on the postsynaptic cells, the question of the nature of the relationship between interneuronal and principal cell parameter variability needs to be addressed. The exact answer to this question is not known, partly because most previous experimental studies did not pay close attention to separating the two cardinal aspects of heterogeneity (i.e., the intragroup variance and between-group species diversity). In fact, there are no solid data even on the fundamental question of whether the interneuronal variability (cell-to-cell variability within a single interneuronal subtype) is actually larger than pyramidal cell variability (note that, as far as cellular species diversity is concerned, there is general agreement that the interneurons as a whole are more diverse than the excitatory cell group).

However, it is important to emphasize that cell-to-cell variability also exists between excitatory cells as well, even if they belong to a seemingly homogeneous population (e.g., CA1 pyramidal cells). As discussed by Somogyi and Klausberger (2005), there may in fact be at least three subpopulations of CA1 pyramidal cells: (1) smaller, weakly calbindin-immunoreactive pyramidal cells in the compact main cell body layer next to the stratum radiatum; (2) larger, more loosely arranged, calbindin-negative pyramidal cells within the cell layer toward the stratum oriens (Baimbridge & Miller, 1982); and (3) pyramidal cells in the stratum radiatum (Maccaferri & McBain, 1996; Gulyás et al., 1998), which may be projecting to the accessory olfactory bulb (Van Groen & Wyss, 1990).

Evidence for certain degree of heterogeneity among CA1 pyramidal cells was also obtained recently by laser capture microdissection in combination with microarrays, a modern combination of techniques that allows the analysis of the expression of thousands of genes in selected cells (Kamme et al., 2003; note that we will discuss these results further in chapter 7). Figure 6.9 illustrates that there were differences in gene expression even among the supposedly homogenous group of CA1 pyramidal cells. However, the gene expression differences were not as pronounced as those seen between pyramidal cells and interneurons. Importantly, clustering results shown in Fig. 6.9 also illustrate that several genes were found clustered in the same group (i.e., they covaried), indicating that the apparent heterogeneity between the CA1 pyramidal cells were not due to a random event. These findings support earlier studies that described that neurons in vivo and in vitro exhibited differences in gene expression among single cells within a given cell type (Mackler et al., 1992; Sheng et al., 1995; Zawar et al., 1999). The differences between individual cells may be caused by purely stochastic processes (Elowitz et al., 2002), but the nonrandom differences indicated by the covaried expression patterns suggest that the cell-to-cell differences may correspond to different functional states, such as participation in field coding, which, in turn, may be related to differences afferent inputs or projection targets (Kamme et al., 2003). Indeed, it has been shown that selected CA1 cells respond to spatial experiences of the rat by changes in gene expression (Guzowski et al., 1999). It is also possible that the cell-to-cell variability among the interneurons is at least partially responsible for the cell-to-cell heterogeneity among the principal cells as well (and the reverse may also apply). In addition, perhaps the fact that only a relatively low number of interneurons belonging to the same subtype converge onto a single pyramidal cell (e.g., about 25 basket cells innervate a

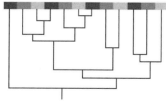

IX _ = VI III x X̄ ≥ V VII > X̄

Rat ATP synthase subunit D mRNA, D13120
AA818688 similar to mouse AA 386997
AA900092 similar to mouse AA369788
Rat 70 kd heat shock-like protein mRNA, M11942
Rat H(+)-transporting ATPase mRNA, AA858959
AA817769 similar to mouse AA183125
Rat t complex polypeptide 1 (Tcp-1) mRNA, D90345
Rat alpha-fodrin (A2A) mRNA, AI030460
EST AA817739
Rat cytochrome C oxidase subunit VIa mRNA, AA955550
AA899459 similar to mouse AA521623
Rat non-neuronal enolase (NNE) mRNA, AA900146
Rat GAPDH mRNA, X02231
Rat cofilin mRNA, AA 859476
Rat polyubiquitin mRNA, AA875068
AA924126 similar to human Sp3 protein mRNA
Rat prenylated rab acceptor 1 (PRA1) mRNA, AA956771
AA899249 similar to mouse AA117876

Figure 6.9   **A cluster indicating differences in gene expression among the pyramidal neurons.** The column dendrogram splits the cells in two major groups, in addition to the interneuron (cell no. IX). The fact that genes are found clustered within groups indicates that they covaried, suggesting that the pyramidal cell heterogeneity may not be due to a random event. Adapted, with permission, from Kamme et al. (2003).

single pyramidal cell in the hippocampus) (Buhl et al., 1994a) may also be important, by leading to stochastic effects and amplifying the differences between pyramidal cells innervated by only partially over-lapping pools of presynaptic interneurons.

Heterogeneity in the Outside World and Its Reflection in the Circuit

If the cell-to-cell heterogeneity in neuronal populations is altered by internal factors such as the neuromodulatory pathways, possibly in a brain state–dependent manner, perhaps heterogeneity may also be modulated by the animal's environment. Currently, this issue is largely unexplored experimentally. However, it is a promising development that new techniques, such as the above-mentioned laser capture microdissection method in combination with microarray analysis (Kamme et al., 2004) provides high-throughput methods with which the question of the environmental regulation of cell-to-cell variability can begin to be addressed in a quantitative, objective manner. For example, would environmental enrichment increase or decrease cell-to-cell variance in an interneuronal population?

This issue is particularly relevant to interneuron research, as virtually all investigations into interneuronal functions are carried out on rats that are raised in standard laboratory cages. Is it possible that some of the cases of apparently unusually high levels of variability in interneuronal properties are at least partly due to the environment in which the rats were raised? For example, could it be that the occasionally observed, unusually high proportion (around 10%) of non-initial segment targets of axo-axonic cells is due to some poorly understood environmental effects, for example, laboratory rats raised in sensorily deprived environment (Somogyi & Klausberger, 2005)? Although no solid answers are yet available, the fact that we now at least begin to ponder these questions, together with the availability of the appropriate statistical approaches to test for the equality of variances discussed above, indicate that precise determination of environmental influences on interneuronal cell-to-cell variability within defined populations will be obtained in the future. We will return to this issue later in the book, when the question of modulation of intraspecies variability and species diversity can be addressed jointly.

Variations for the Advanced Age: Intraspecies Variance in Interneuronal Populations through Somatic Mutations?

In the preceding discussions on the possible sources of intra-subtype variance, the emphasis was placed on alterations in gene expression levels. This focus is a natural consequence of the widely held assumption that cells, neuronal or non-neuronal, in the body all share the same genetic material. However, it has been known for some time that somatic mutations (i.e., mutations in non-germline cells) can occur, and recent data suggest that the extent and rate of somatic mutations may not be as rare as previously assumed.

Mutation load, the frequency of each type of mutation, appears to increase with age and to be tissue specific. A variety of genetic modifications undergoes increases with age (Hill et al., 2004), including sister chromatid exchange (Schneider et al., 1979), chromosome loss (Fenech, 1998), micronuclei (Dass et al., 1997; Bolognesi et al., 1999), chromosomal aberrations (Mukherjee & Thomas, 1997; Bolognesi et al., 1999), single-strand DNA breaks (Chetsanga et al., 1977; Ono et al., 1995) and rearrangements, point mutations, deletions, and insertions (Buettner et al., 1999; Dolle et al., 2000; Ono et al., 2000; Stuart et al., 2000). Mutation load assessments based on endogenous gene targets are limited to a few genes in a few cell types. For example, the frequency of human hypoxanthine phosphoribosyl transferase (HPRT) mutants increases with age (Robinson et al., 1994; Curry et al., 1999). In contrast, mutation detection systems based on transgenic mice can identify mutations in practically any tissue and cell type. In these transgenic systems, mice carry a chromosomally integrated lambda bacteriophage containing the *Escherichia coli* LacI or lacZ gene as a target for mutagenesis (Kohler et al., 1991; Gossen et al., 1989). These two transgenic systems are referred to as the Big Blue and Muta mouse systems, respectively. The Big Blue system, in particular, has an extensive database (de Boer & Glickman, 1998) and is well validated (Hill et al., 1999). A recent study using this system showed that the mutation frequency (determined by dividing the number of mutant blue plaques by the total number of screened plaques on dilution plates as described in the Big Blue protocol by Stratagene) shows tissue-specific time-courses during aging, but similar mutation types (Hill et al., 2004). By definition, somatic mutation load is zero at conception, which is followed by an early rapid phase of spontaneous mutagenesis. Intriguingly, mutation frequencies at 10 days in mice were higher in the forebrain (2.1×10^{-5}) and cerebellum (2.7×10^{-5}) than in liver and thymus (both 1.6×10^{-5}). However, there was no further increase in mutation frequencies with old age in the neuronal structures in the latter study (but see below). The finding that the spectrum of mutation types showed less variation than mutation frequency raised the interesting but unresolved question of whether mutation rates and types would be drastically different in cell types that produce substantial amounts of mutagenic products, such as intracellular nitric oxide (which may be generated in certain nitric oxide synthase–positive interneurons) and hydrogen peroxide (dopaminergic neurons generate one such molecule for every neurotransmitter molecule synthesized; Ischiropoulos et al., 1992).

What is the aggregate functional effect of these apparently low mutation rates? In fact, most murine systems, regardless of a number of potentially confounding factors (e.g., transgene integration site, copy number, genetic background, somatic tissue types), show rather similar mutation rates to those cited above, with only a few mutants per 100,000 targets screened (Zhang et al., 1995; Swiger et al., 1999, 2001). It should also be noted that if the average mutation is recessive, in animals with diploid cells, most cells would stay relatively unaffected, as the second copy of the gene on the other chromosome would permit normal function (Driver, 2004). In addition, although the transgenes are useful surrogates for mutational studies, several of their characteristics may not be identical to those of endogenous loci. Thus, albeit these studies point to somatic mutations, and indicate the role of general metabolism and reactive oxygen species as major components of aging, they do not resolve the key issue of interest to us, (i.e., the effect of these somatic mutations on individual interneurons in specific cortical areas and their contribution to intraspecies interneuronal variance).

Nevertheless, there are some intriguing new data that suggest that the role of somatic mutations may be quite important in the brain. First, it has been pointed out that although the individual acquired somatic mutations may not achieve high mutational burdens in the brain, the cumulative effects of multiple individually rare mutations may be significant (Simon et al., 2004). Second, mutations could take place not only in the nuclear DNA, but also in the mitochondrial DNA (mtDNA). Given the key role of mitochondrial metabolism in normal cell life, it is significant that the most mtDNA damage does occur in the brain and the heart, tissues with high rates of oxidative metabolism (Kovalenko et al., 1998).

A recent study presented a real breakthrough in our understanding of the alterations in gene regulation and DNA damage in the aging human brain (Lu et al., 2004). These authors examined frontal cortical samples in persons aged from 26 to 106 years using Affymetrix gene chips. Using this technology, it was possible to screen about 11,000 genes, and about 4% of these showed significant changes with age. Importantly, the microarray data were validated by comparisons with real-time polymerase chain reaction (PCR) results for a subset of the genes, and the data were also consistent with alterations in protein levels assessed with Western blotting. In addition, the alterations in gene expressions were not likely to be associated with major changes in cell numbers, as a number of neuron-specific markers, including β-tubulin, GAP-43, and syntaxin-1, did not change significantly with age. The findings showed a cluster of genes that were downregulated and another cluster that was upregulated. The downregulated genes included a number of genes that play roles in learning and synaptic plasticity, memory storage and long-term potentiation (LTP), including the synaptic calcium signaling system, which may be relevant for the age-related changes in cognitive functions. Although some of the alterations involved genes that are not expressed in cortical GABAergic neurons (e.g., CAM kinase II), others clearly could involve interneuronal systems. These latter genes included somatostatin, calbindin, and calretinin, which all showed about a twofold decrease. In addition, the β3 subunit of the GABA$_A$ receptor displayed a large, threefold drop in expression with age. Thus, there is little doubt that GABAergic systems, including key molecules involved in interneuronal calcium homeostasis and GABAergic transmission, are significantly altered with age.

The cluster of genes that showed increased expressions included genes that mediate the stress responses and repair, which led to the hypothesis that oxidative DNA damage might specifically target promoter regions containing (G+C)-rich sequences (these are sensitive to oxidative damage and are not repaired by transcription-coupled processes). Indeed, DNA damage appeared in many genes after age 40, and, astonishingly, DNA damage was pervasive in virtually all the examined genes by age 70 (Lu et al., 2004). Therefore, oxidative damage that may arise from mitochondria targets selectively vulnerable genes involved in learning and memory, resulting in downregulation of these genes, but also leading to the upregulation of antioxidant enzymes and DNA repair genes. These data from the normal human aging brains were complemented and enlarged by recent findings that certain somatic mtDNA control-region mutations were present in a very high percent (65%) of Alzheimer brains (Coskun et al., 2004), far exceeding the control rates.

Taken together, these results show that somatic mutations in the brain may be more frequent than previously believed, and they may result in substantial alterations in synaptic functions involved in learning and memory (i.e., they may have behaviorally significant effects even at the whole organism level). Furthermore, the alterations in the expression levels of genes in cortical tissues that are expressed in interneurons and at GABAergic synapses, including somatostatin, calbindin, and certain $GABA_A$ receptor subunits, indicate that these complex processes may contribute to age-dependent changes in cell-to-cell variance within interneuronal populations. In this context, it is also noteworthy that DNA damage is markedly increased specifically in the promoters of genes with decreased expressions in the aged cortical tissues, which, therefore, likely include interneuron-related gene promoters as well. Given the apparent connection between metabolic and mutation rates, it is interesting to consider that interneurons, and especially the fast-spiking basket cells, are likely to be among the most metabolically active neurons in the brain, as indicated by their high firing rates and the presence of large and numerous mitochondria. Combinations of various techniques, including the Big Blue mouse model in conjunction with the gene chips approaches, could offer key insights into the issue of somatic mutation rates and DNA damage in specific promoter regions in interneuronal subtypes at various developmental time-points.

7

Diversity Beyond Variance

> *Up to this point I have spoken of the measure of diversity only as the number of species: so many bacteria in a pinch of soil, so many ants in a stretch of rain forest. What also matters very much is the relative abundance of species.*
>
> Edward O. Wilson (1992)

Species Number and Relative Abundance: Entropy-Based Measures of Diversity

The measures of intraspecies parameter variance discussed in the previous chapter cannot be readily applied to the entirely different problem of quantification of interneuronal species diversity. The ideal diversity measure should be able to reflect the diversity of interneuronal species in at least two fundamental ways (Földy et al., 2005). First, it should take into account how many species make up a particular network, as most researchers would agree that a network with more interneuronal species is more diverse. However, a second aspect is the relative abundance of the species. Intuitively, most of us would agree that a network where all interneuronal species are found at exactly the same rate is more diverse than a network where certain species are abundant but others are exceedingly rare (Wilson, 1992). This is because each interneuron that we encounter is less predictable in a more diverse system, and thus it gives us more information on average (Földy et al., 2005).

The problem of a lack of a well-defined approach to measuring diversity is especially evident when it comes to addressing changes in interneuronal species diversity during development or in neurological diseases. Changes in diversity may take place in neurological disorders such as trauma, ischemia, or epilepsy, accompanied by the complete or partial loss of specific interneuronal classes, leading to alterations in the number and relative abundance of distinct interneuronal species (Santhakumar & Soltesz, 2004). So the question is how does interneuronal diversity change, in precise, quantitative terms, if a specific type of interneuron is selectively lost from the network following an insult? Does interneuronal diversity decrease more when a rare interneuronal class is lost, compared to the loss of a relatively abundant type? How does diversity change when a previously unified interneuronal group is divided into two (e.g., after the discovery of a novel, functionally relevant marker)? In general, what measure of diversity should one use to quantify interneuronal diversity in a particular neuronal network and its changes after various manipulations?

An insight into these questions came from a recent study that employed the Shannon–Wiener diversity index to the problem of interneuronal diversity (Földy et al., 2004). This particular measure of diversity is used in other disciplines; for example, it is used to assess the number and relative abundance of animal and plant species in ecosystem studies (Wilson & Bossert 1971), and it is also widely used in information theory and neuronal coding (Dayan & Abbott 2001).

The Shannon–Wiener diversity index is defined as

$$D = -\sum_{i=1}^{k} p_i \log p_i$$

where k is the number of categories, and p_i is the proportion of observations in category i (Zar, 1999). The measure D is formally equivalent to entropy, and it is a dimensionless number that describes how "interesting" or "surprising" a set of events (observations) is. For a single category (when there is only a single cellular species present in the network), the diversity index is zero (D = 0), and for two or more subgroups, D increases (Földy et al., 2004, 2005). D takes different values for different distributions (e.g., a uniform distribution where all events occur with the same probability vs. a Gaussian distribution). Although here we emphasized interneuronal species diversity, it is important to recognize that categories used to compute the diversity index can be either synaptic or cellular; for example, they can be the G_{IPSC} values that can occur. Note that the diversity indices established for different parameters are additive.

Plasticity of Interneuronal Diversity: Birth and Loss of Cellular Species

The actual diversity index value for the various parameters of GABAergic systems in cortical microcircuits is only beginning to be assessed. Table 7.1 illustrates, in a step-by-step fashion, the details of its calculation for the interneuronal species that are present in the rat dentate gyrus (Santhakumar & Soltesz, 2004; Földy et al., 2005). The precise assessment of D values in various cortical areas in normal, healthy situations will be extremely useful for determining, in precise terms, the fundamental, quantitative features of interneuronal diversity. In addition, the application of the Shannon–Wiener diversity index to various neurological disease paradigms is promising to be a uniquely useful, simple tool to express pathological changes in interneuronal species diversity in quantitative terms. Figure 7.1 illustrates the alterations in diversity index values of

Table 7.1   Step-by-step calculation of the interneuronal diversity index for the interneuronal network of the dentate gyrus.

Interneuron Species	k	$p_i = \dfrac{n}{total}$	$p_i \log p_i$
PV+ Basket Cell	1	$\dfrac{12000}{44000} = 0.2727$	−0.1539
CCK+ Basket Cell	2	0.1818	−0.1346
HIPP Cell	3	0.2727	−0.1539
MOPP Cell	4	0.0909	−0.0947
HICAP Cell	5	0.0682	−0.0795
IS Cell	6	0.0682	−0.0795
Axo-Axonic Cell	7	0.0455	−0.0610
$D = -\sum\limits_{i=1}^{k} p_i \log p_i \rightarrow$			$D = 0.7571$

PV+, parvalbumin-positive; CCK+, cholecystokinin-positive; HIPP and MOPP cells, Hilar or molecular layer cells, respectively, with axonal projections to the part of the molecular layer innervated by the perforant path; HICAP cells, Hilar cells with axonal projections to the associational pathway (inner molecular layer); IS cells, interneuron-specific cells. For values of n (total number of cells of a particular species), see Fig. 7.1.
Reprinted, with permission, from Földy et al. (2005).

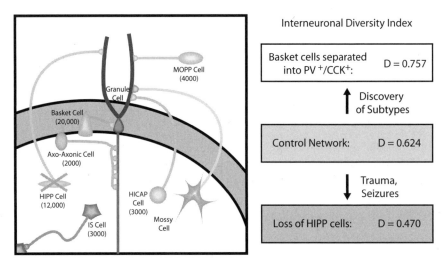

Figure 7.1   **Quantification of interneuronal diversity in control and pathological states.**
The figure illustrates changes in the diversity index (D) for interneurons in the control
dentate gyrus, after the loss of a particular interneuronal population (loss of HIPP cells
after trauma and seizures) and after the subdivision of a previously unified cell class
(illustrated by the separation of basket cells into PV$^+$ and CCK$^+$ subpopulations).
Excitatory granule cells and mossy cells are also illustrated, but they are not included in
the calculation of the interneuronal diversity index. Number of parvalbumin-positive
basket cells: 12,000; cholecystokinin-positive basket cells: 8,000. For abbreviations for the
cell types, see Table 7.1. Note that the exact nature of the postsynaptic targets of IS cells
are not fully known, so the IS cell is only connected to one other IS cell for simplicity).
Adapted, with permission, from Santhakumar et al. (2004).

control and injured interneuronal networks of the dentate gyrus.
The diversity index of the control network decreased after the loss of
a vulnerable hilar interneuronal cell type. Note that, in contrast, the
diversity index would increase if a previously homogeneous interneuronal population is subdivided into two distinct subpopulations.
Both the cell loss–induced decrease and the subdivision-related
increase in the diversity index correlate well with commonsense
notions about changes in cellular diversity after decreases and
increases in species number.

     Note that there are many neurobiologically relevant situations
where the interneuronal diversity may change, and, consequently,
where application of the above-defined diversity index will be
extremely beneficial to quantitatively address modifications in
interneuronal diversity. In chapter 2, we discussed how the distant

site of interneuron generation during development likely makes the developmental processes (e.g., migration) of these cells especially sensitive to various modulatory influences and vulnerable to environmental disruptions, which may result in alterations in either species numbers (e.g., loss of a particular interneuronal subtype) or in relative abundance (e.g., changes in the number of individuals of a particular interneuronal species), both of which would be reflected in a modified diversity index. Quantification of interneuronal diversity would make it possible to precisely determine the relative magnitude of the effects of various developmental disturbances or insults on the cellular composition of the adult neuronal network. As Fig. 7.1 illustrates, certain interneuronal species are especially vulnerable to insults, particularly in the dentate hilus. In general, dendritically projecting interneurons are often reported to be more sensitive than perisomatically projecting cells in many seizure and trauma paradigms (Toth et al., 1997a; Cossart et al., 2001). Within the perisomatically projecting populations, the CCK-positive basket cells appear to be more prone to undergo pathological forms of plasticity than parvalbumin-containing cells (Freund, 2003; Chen et al., 2003; Sayin et al., 2003). Although the array of selective vulnerability patterns for interneurons is certainly large, it is possible that the many faces of selective vulnerability may reflect the multiple distinct mechanisms that underlie neuronal injury and death. For example, immediately after concussive head trauma, a highly selective initial pattern of injury emerges among interneuronal populations for purely mechanical reasons (Toth et al., 1997a), related to cell size and the cell type specific expression of cytoskeletal elements providing structural support (Ratzliff and Soltesz, 2000, 2001). Subsequently, this initial pattern of injury is then modified further in specific ways by biological (e.g., glutamatergic excitotoxic) mechanisms, which may be a key factor in deciding whether a cell that was injured during the initial impact dies or survives long-term (Toth et al., 1997a). Again, application of the diversity index will allow the precise measurement of the changes in interneuronal species diversity in each of the various, distinct steps identified during the progression of a neurological dieases (e.g., the "latent period" after the initial insult, followed by the appearance of full-blown, recurrent seizures in many models of temporal lobe epilepsy) (e.g., Coulter, 2001; Dyhrfjeld-Johnsen & Soltesz, 2004; Shah et al. 2004).

Finally, it should be mentioned that a new dimension for plasticity of interneuronal diversity may arise from the generation of newly born cells (Santhakumar & Soltesz, 2004). In addition to the continued neurogenesis of granule cells in the adult dentate gyrus (Markakis & Gage, 1999), there is recent evidence that interneurons may also be among the newly generated neurons. GABAergic precursor cells have been reported to exist in the adult dentate gyrus, as shown by the ability of endogenous stem cells isolated from the adult hippocampus to give rise to functional GABAergic inhibitory cells in culture (Takahashi et al., 1999). In addition, a considerable number of the newly generated cells in the dentate gyrus appeared to include interneurons, with most of the new GABAergic cells being immunoreactive for parvalbumin (Liu et al., 2003). The newly generated cells evoked fast unitary IPSCs in granule cells in simultaneous paired recordings (Liu et al., 2003), indicating the ability of the younger interneurons to integrate synaptically into the dentate circuit. In light of reports that seizures and trauma can dramatically enhance the rate of granule cell generation (Parent et al., 1997; Dash et al., 2001; Yoshimura et al., 2001), it is an intriguing possibility, to be determined in future studies, that the birth rate of new interneurons may also be altered after insults. Such a change in birth rate would be expected to also alter the Shannon–Wiener diversity index, even if no new interneuronal species are generated.

Effects of Changed Diversity on Firing Rates

How do alterations in diversity modulate neuronal functions? As discussed in chapters 5 and 6, computational and experimental studies (Aradi & Soltesz, 2002; Aradi et al., 2002, 2004) showed that the effects of heterogeneous, perisomatic populations of G_{IPSC}s on the average firing rate of the postsynaptic cell depended on the mean of the G_{IPSC} peak amplitude (or decay), the variance in the G_{IPSC} peak amplitude (or decay), the excitation that the postsynaptic cell received, and on E_{GABA}. Furthermore, it was also discussed in chapter 5 how the variance-effects crucially depended on the the position of the "critical region." Here we will show that the simple rules outlined in chapter 5 for the variance-effects can be applied to changes in diversity as well. Therefore, here we investigate the impact of GABAergic heterogeneity not through changes in variance, but through alterations in diversity, defined as the number and relative abundance of subgroups within a G_{IPSC} population, and quantified using the Shannon–Wiener diversity index (Földy et al., 2004).

Figure 7.2 illustrates how increasing diversity (represented by the increasing number of subgroups) can be predicted (for simplicity, only the case of a broad distribution such as b in Fig. 7.2A around B_1 is explained below, but the same logic can be applied to any mean and standard variation) (Földy et al., 2004). If the mean G_{IPSC} is smaller than (but close to) the critical region (B_1 in Fig. 7.2A), a homogenous G_{IPSC} group (i.e., SD = 0) will let the cell fire with a certain rate (f_{max} in Figs. 7.2B and 7.2D; the actual value of f_{max} depends on the amount of depolarizing current that the cell receives). Increasing the number of subgroups from one to two (symmetrically around B_1) is expected to decrease the average firing rate, as the variance is high enough for the larger subgroup to fall to the right of the critical region. Increasing the number of subgroups from two to three (while keeping the mean and SD the same) is expected to decrease the proportion of the events that fall to the right of the critical region (as now one G_{IPSC} subgroup equals B_1, one is smaller than B_1, and only one subgroup is larger than B_1), therefore, the average firing rate is predicted to increase from the lower levels reached with two subgroups, but still stay below f_{max} (Fig. 1D, filled circles labeled "1" through "3"). Similarly, increasing the number of G_{IPSC} subgroups from three to four is expected to produce two subgroups (Fig. 7.2C) that are larger than the critical region, which is predicted to decrease the average firing rate, as illustrated in Fig. 7.2D (filled circle labeled "4"). In the limit, when the number of subgroups approaches infinity, we have a continuous distribution (Fig. 7.2C), and the effect on the firing rate can be predicted as described above in connection with the variance effects (Figs. 7.2A and 7.2B). Note that when the mean value is larger than the critical region (B_2 in Fig. 7.2A), then increasing diversity increases the firing frequency (open circles in Fig. 7.2D). Because it is not simply the number of subgroups that determines the diversity effects, but also the relative frequency of occurrence of the events within the various subgroups, we use the diversity index as the independent variable in both the simulation and the dynamic clamp studies designed to test the predictions outlined above.

Figure 7.3 shows that the predictions illustrated in Fig. 7.2D were confirmed by the computational and dynamic clamp experiments.

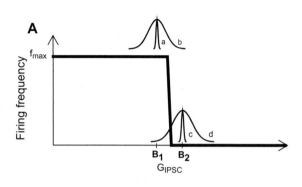

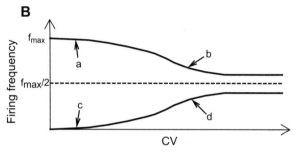

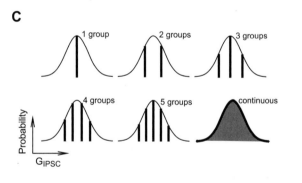

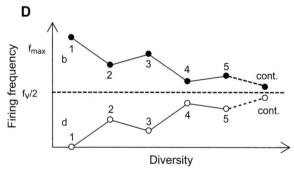

First, the predicted effects of altered diversity were tested in model CA1 pyramidal cells. G_{IPSC}s were injected into the cell around the experimentally observed mIPSC peak G_{IPSC} mean and SD (Földy et al., 2004), using a uniform distribution for simplicity (i.e., the events occurred in a random order but with equal probability within each subgroup; Gaussian distribution gave similar results; the cells were depolarized with a certain amount of depolarizing current so that the cell discharged at around 15–20 Hz with G_{IPSC} = 0). When all G_{IPSC}s were exactly the same ("normalized diversity" = D = 0 in Fig. 7.3A), increasing the G_{IPSC}s (along the x axis labeled "G_{IPSC}") resulted in an input–output function similar to that described in Fig. 7.2A. As expected, when the diversity was increased (along the z axis labeled "normalized diversity" in Fig. 7.3A) from a single group to two and more groups, the average firing rate showed prominent changes only if the mean G_{IPSC}s were close to the critical region. If the mean G_{IPSC} was smaller than the critical region, increasing D first caused a decrease, then a relative increase in the firing rate (thick line in Fig. 7.3A, shown in detail in Fig. 7.3B with examples of the conductance commands and the firing activity), as predicted in

---

Figure 7.2 **Predictions of the effects of changes in input heterogeneity on firing rates.** Panels A and B show the variance effects (Aradi et al., 2002; see also Fig. 5.8), whereas panels C and D illustrate the diversity effects (Földy et al., 2004). (A) Schematic drawing of an input–output plot (thick line), indicating the effects of populations of G_{IPSC}s with CV = 0 on the postsynaptic cell's firing rates (note that the cell fires tonically when G_{IPSC} = 0, as a result of a depolarizing current input). The sharp drop in firing rate is referred to as the "critical region." Note that B1 is the mean of distributions "a" and "b," whereas B2 represents the mean of distributions "c" and "d." (B) When the cell is challenged with populations of G_{IPSC}s that have a nonzero CV (indicated by the Gaussian distributions labelled "a" through "d" above the input–output plot in A), the resulting changes in firing rates can be predicted as indicated by the letters a–d corresponding to the distributions in A. (C) Schematic drawings of the subgroups that can have the same population mean and variance as a Gaussian (as long as the number of subgroups is >1, as with a single group the variance is zero). The most diverse distribution is the continuous distribution (infinite number of subgroups). (D) Predictions of the effects of increasing diversity (defined based on the number and relative abundance of subgroups) on firing rates. Filled circles indicate the expected plot when the mean is smaller than the critical region (e.g., distribution "b" from panel A), whereas the open circles indicate the predictions when the distribution mean is larger than the critical region (distribution "d" in panel A). The numbers next to the symbols refer to the number of subgroups indicated in panel C. Note the characteristic up-down-up (or down-up-down) pattern of the modulation of firing rates by the increasing diversity index. Reprinted, with permission, from Földy et al. (2004).

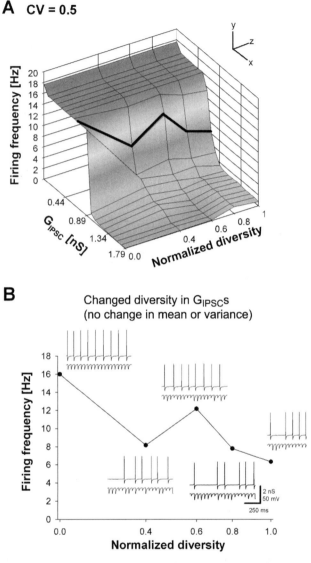

A CV = 0.5

B Changed diversity in G_{IPSC}s
(no change in mean or variance)

Figure 7.3 **Modulation of firing rates by diversity in peak G_{IPSC} in model CA1 pyramidal cells.** (A) Three-dimensional plot shows the effects of increasing mean G_{IPSC}s (on the x axis; see inset for axes orientations), and of increasing diversity (along the z axis), on the firing rate (on the y axis). The cell received a certain amount of depolarizing current so that it discharged around 15–20 Hz (I_{depol} = 0.13 nA), and that the critical region was close to the experimentally determined miniature IPSC mean$_{exp}$ and SD$_{exp}$ peak G_{IPSC} values. A uniform distribution was used for generating G_{IPSC}s with various mean and diversity values. The x–y plane at zero diversity shows the effects of increasing mean G_{IPSC} without variance. Note that the SD values were adjusted when the means were changed

Fig. 7.2D (filled circles). In contrast, there was little effect of changing diversity when D was increased around mean G_{IPSC} values that were far from the critical value. As could be predicted from the simple rules explained in connection with Fig. 7.2, decreasing the scatter around the mean (from $CV_{exp} = 0.5$ to $CV = 0.25$) also decreased the effects of increasing D on average firing rates. Similarly to the G_{IPSC} peak amplitude diversity, the modulation of firing rates by diversity in G_{IPSC} frequency was also shown to conform to the predictions (Földy et al., 2004). Furthermore, just like with the variance-effects, the computational modeling results on the effects of diversity in peak G_{IPSC}s and frequency could also be replicated in biological CA1 pyramidal cells using dynamic clamping (Földy et al., 2004).

Taken together, these results show that changes in the diversity index of GABAergic inhibitory synaptic events can exert significant effects on the firing rates, even if the mean and variance of the event amplitude and frequency do not change.

Modulation of Synchrony by Alterations in Diversity

In the preceding section, GABAergic synaptic event diversity was examined. The studies discussed above allowed us to demonstrate, in relatively simple, easily understandable situations, how event group number and relative abundance can modulate neuronal activity. However, although synaptic groupings may originate from distinct interneuronal classes, they do not readily translate to interneuronal species diversity. Therefore, we now continue our discussion by examining the effects of altering diversity in a network model of

---

so that CV remained the same ($CV_{exp} = 0.5$). As expected, increasing diversity at this CV had strong effects on firing rates only when the mean G_{IPSC} was close to the critical region. (B) The thick line in panel A is shown in detail with example traces for the conductance commands (bottom traces) and the cell's response (upper traces). Note that the starting point (at D = 0) was to the left of the critical region (i.e., the G_{IPSC} mean around which the diversity was introduced was too small to cause suppression of firing when diversity was zero) therefore as predicted, increasing diversity first decreases, then relatively enhances, then again decreases the firing rate. For D-effects at various CVs, see Földy et al. (2004). E_{GABA} was set to –65 mV. Adapted, with permission, from Földy et al. (2004).

interneurons on network coherence (i.e., on synchrony of firing). Because of its importance and heuristic value, the modulation of network synchrony by interneuronal diversity will be discussed in detail below. Note that these effects occurred without concurrent changes in means or variances.

The interneuronal subgroups, for simplicity, differed only in a single parameter, in the amount of excitation that they received (Földy et al., 2004) (note that real interneurons can also exhibit marked differences in the amount of glutamatergic synapses on their dendrites, e.g., in the case of PV^+ vs. CCK^+ interneurons; see chapter 3). The simulation results (Földy et al., 2004, 2005) are shown in Fig. 7.4. The population consisted of either n = 12 or n = 120 cells (the interneurons had a single compartment and were identical, and connected in an all to all pattern), and the networks were divided into 1 to 6 groups (G_{syn} was 0.015 nS for the 12-cell network, and it was adjusted to 0.0015 nS for the 120-cell network, in order to preserve the total synaptic input strength per cell). Synchrony was measured as "coherence," following White et al. (1998). As mentioned above, cellular diversity was simulated by the introduction of distinct amounts of I_{depol} that the cells received. Importantly, in order to be able to study the effects of altered diversity alone, without confounding changes in mean and variance, the different depolarizing current values were distributed according to a uniform distribution so that the mean I_{depol} = 0.6 nA and the SD I_{depol} = 0.115 nA were unchanged as diversity increased (with the exception of the case of D = 0, when, because there is only a single group, SD = 0). Before the effects of diversity on coherence were studied, it was determined in a separate series of simulations that increasing SD among cells in I_{depol} (between 0 nA to 0.34 nA around mean I_{depol} = 0.6 nA) did indeed cause the expected, and previously demonstrated, decrease in coherence (Golomb & Rinzel, 1993; Wang & Buzsáki, 1996; White et al., 1998; Aradi & Soltesz, 2002) (discussed in chapter 5).

For the sake of simplicity and easier understanding, the results concerning three groups are first explained in detail for the 12-cell network and illustrated by the raster plots in Fig. 7.4 (Földy et al., 2004, 2005). As an initial step, the discharge rate of interneurons were first determined when all 12 cells received the same I_{depol} (i.e., D = 0), first 0.84 nA, then 0.6 nA, and finally 0.35 nA. Because the diversity was zero in each simulation, the cells discharged in

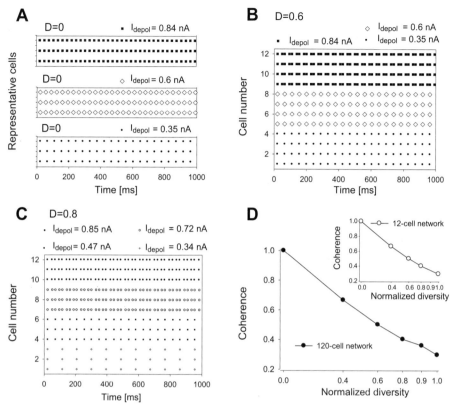

Figure 7.4 **Modulation of network coherence by interneuronal diversity.** (A) Raster plots illustrate the effects of three different I_{depol} values on a 12-cell network. In each group, diversity (D) was set to 0, and all the 12 cells received the same I_{depol} value (0.35, 0.6, or 0.84 nA). The firing of three out of the 12 cells from each case is illustrated. In (B), the diversity was introduced in the depolarizing current that the cells received (a uniform distribution was used). The 12 cells were subdivided into three groups, with each subgroup receiving a different amount of I_{depol} (the I_{depol} values were the same as in A). Note that the cell subgroup that received the largest amount of I_{depol} enhanced its firing rate (top group), whereas the middle subgroup slowed down. (C) Raster plot shows the firing of four subgroups (D = 0.8). (D) Plot of the network coherence (White et al., 1998) as a function of the normalized diversity index (D = 1 is for six subgroups) for the 120-cell network (G_{syn} = 0.0015 nS). Note the decrease in coherence with increasing diversity. Also note that diversity modulated network coherence even though the mean and CV for the whole population did not change (mean I_{depol} = 0.6 nA; CV = 0.115). The inset shows similar results for the 12-cell network used for the explanations in the text for simplicity. Reprinted, with permission, from Földy et al. (2004).

complete synchrony in all three cases (3 out of the 12 cells from each of the three simulations are illustrated in Fig. 7.4A). As expected, the interneurons discharged at the highest rate when they received the strongest depolarizing current (top three cells in Fig. 7.4A), but the difference between the firing rates with the three I_{depol} values was relatively small (range, 35 Hz to 22.5 Hz; firing rate of the 12 identical cells with the different I_{depol} values: with 0.84 nA, 35 Hz; with 0.6 nA, 29 Hz; with 0.35 nA, 22.5 Hz). The reason for the relatively small difference in firing rates with the different I_{depol} values was that, as the interneurons increased their firing rates with a stronger I_{depol}, they received a stronger inhibition from the other cells, which also received a similarly strong excitation (Földy et al., 2004).

As the next step, the cellular diversity in the population was increased by dividing the 12 cells into three groups, with each group receiving a different I_{depol} at the same time (either 0.84 nA, or 0.6 nA, or 0.35 nA). Increasing the diversity in this way (to D = 0.6) resulted in a robust separation of the firing rates of the three subgroups of cells (but the cells within each subgroup still fired in synchrony). The subgroup that received the strongest I_{depol} (cells 9 to 12 in Fig. 7.4B, receiving I_{depol} = 0.84 nA) increased their firing rates to 44.5 Hz, whereas the middle subgroup slowed down to the rate of the slowest subgroup (to 22.5 Hz).

In other words, the interneuronal subgroup receiving the strongest excitation suppressed the other cells and decreased their firing rates, simultaneously increasing its own discharge rate (since it received less inhibition, due to the decreased discharge rate in the inhibited cells) (Földy et al., 2004). Therefore, in a sense, this is a "rich get richer" scheme, where the interneurons that receive the strongest excitation fire faster because of the higher degree of depolarization and also because they depress firing in the other groups.

As a result of the segregation in the relative firing rates between the groups, an increase in the number of groups strongly modulated network coherence (Figs. 7.4B–7.4D; the raster plot in Fig. 7.4C shows the case for 4 groups, D = 0.8). As diversity in the interneuronal network became larger and larger, the network coherence decreased (Fig. 7.4D, inset). Note that the group that discharged at the slowest rate still fired phased-locked with the other groups, but the fastest group fired many more times than the slowest group (Fig. 7.4C), resulting in a decrease in the overall network coherence. Similar results were obtained when 120 cells (instead of 12) were implemented in the network (Fig. 7.4D). These simulation results (Földy et al., 2004, 2005) illustrate that interneuron network coherence can show significant alterations with alterations in diversity even if the mean and variance of a parameter (in this case, I_{depol}) are unchanged (Santhakumar & Soltesz, 2004).

Equitability, and Alpha, Beta, and Gamma Diversity

The preceding sections focused on interneuronal diversity as defined and measured by the Shannon–Wiener diversity index. As mentioned above, the diversity index measures not only the number of interneuronal species in a particular network, but it also reflects the relative abundance of the subtypes. A related term for relative abundance is equitability, or the evenness of the abundance of the various interneuronal subtypes. Thus, a network where one interneuronal species is very abundant (e.g., comprising 60% of the individual interneurons) is a network of low equitability. In contrast, a network where each species is represented at a roughly equivalent abundance is a network with high equitability. The diversity index would give the highest value for a network with high equitability (in fact, the highest possible D value would arise when all interneuronal species are represented in equal abundance). It is interesting to point out that the dentate interneuronal network examined above (Table 7.1) has a fairly high equitability, as parvalbumin- and CCK-positive basket cells and HIPP cells are represented in approximately equal abundance, and the rest of the currently known interneuronal species making up the dentate gyrus (the MOPP, HICAP, IS and axo-axonic cells) are still found in reasonable numbers. Of course, it is virtually certain that many more interneuronal species will be defined in the future in the dentate gyrus (similarly to CA1, see Fig. 3.1), either because of the splitting up of an existing species into two or due to the discovery of hitherto unknown, and presumably rare, species.

The possibility for the exact measurement of diversity, provided by the Shannon–Wiener index, may also be extended beyond the interneuronal diversity discussed above, which focused on interneuronal diversity in one particular network, in one specific brain area. Taking cues from ecology, this kind of diversity can be referred to as alpha diversity (Wilson, 1992; Loreau et al., 2001). However, it is clear that diversity, in the common usage of the word among researchers, also reflects differences between brain areas or subdivisions. The second measure of diversity is called beta diversity, which reflects the rate at which the interneuronal species number increases as nearby areas (anatomically defined, distinct neuronal networks) are added. The final diversity measure is the so-called gamma diversity, which accounts for the totality of interneuronal species in all networks in the brain (or in the entire nervous system) of an animal. Currently, we have little information about beta diversity, and our current knowledge is especially spotty about gamma diversity in the case of mammalian brains.

Molecular Dragnets Cast Wide: Interneuronal Species from Unsupervised Clustering

In order to precisely measure interneuronal diversity, especially for beta and gamma diversity, a precise definition of interneuronal species is needed. It is useful to return here to the problem that we already touched upon in chapter 4, that is, that there is no currently available, widely accepted interneuronal species definition. In practice, the axonal target specificity, together with the dendritic characteristics and one or two major immunocytochemical markers are used to define the individual interneuronal subtypes (note that marker-based, essentially "candidate gene" approaches frequently employ in situ hybridization for the marker genes, instead of immunocytochemistry). Of course, a related but unresolved issue is exactly when we consider two interneuronal groups different. Would the differential expression of a single protein define two subtypes? The answer is probably yes, especially if that protein would endow the cells with some distinct functional property. But would we consider two CCK-positive basket cells in two closely related brain areas, say in the dentate gyrus and CA3, different? The answer is probably not, if they express similar immunocytochemical signatures and functional properties in both circuits. But what about basket cells in the dentate gyrus and the cerebellum? Here the answer becomes much more difficult, as we are left with an essentially subjective judgment, due to the lack of a precise definition for the category of interneuronal species. For example, one may argue that cerebellar basket cells are entirely different species, because they, unlike the dentate basket cells, form unique extensions (named "pinceau" or brushes by Cajal) on their terminals that are situated in close proximity, but do not form synapses with, the Purkinje cell axon initial segments (see Howard et al., 2005).

These examples illustrate that there is indeed a strong need for a clear and practical species definition for interneurons. We already discussed (in chapter 4) the limitations of purely anatomical species definitions (e.g., that the same axonal target regions can be shared by otherwise different interneurons), and that it is not clear whether a basket cell should have minimally 20% or 50% of its synapses on somata. How about species definitions that rest upon functional attributes only? Let's consider two function-based species definitions to illustrate their own serious limitations. Here is the first: An individual interneuron belongs to a species if that neuron can functionally substitute for any member of the interneuronal species in question. We all feel, in all likelihood, that this definition grasps an important aspect of what is implicitly meant by species category, however, this definition is not practical (although it could be done in a computational model network), and it is also not entirely clear exactly what functional tests should be used to determine the outcome of the substitution. Note that a reverse definition is also problematic, for exactly the same reasons: An individual interneuron belongs to a species if the deletion of that single neuron from the circuit causes the same functional defect or defects as the deletion of any other member of the interneuronal species in question. So here is completely different, but still essentially functional definition: Interneurons that belong to the same species are connected to each other by gap junctions (Gibson et al., 1999; Galarreta & Hestrin, 1999, 2001; Beierlein et al., 2000; Tamas et al., 2000; Szabadics et al., 2001). This definition, while initially appealing, suffers from several problems. For example, gap junctional connectivity is only preferential between interneurons of the same kind, but it is not absolutely selective, and we are not yet sure if all interneuronal subtypes are indeed connected by gap junctions (although, as discussed in chapter 3, many seem to be). In addition, new results indicate that neurogliaform cells form gap junctions not only with neurogliaform cells, but also with other interneuronal subtypes (Simon et al., 2005).

So let's try the most evident molecular definition: Interneurons belonging to the same species express identical sets of genes. This is a much more appealing definition, mainly because the expression of similar sets of proteins would be expected to endow cells with similar functional properties (but see the next chapter). A major limitation of this definition in practice has been our lack of ability to survey a large number of proteins in single cells (immunocytochemistry is generally limited to only a few proteins at a time). However, with the recent, spectacular advancement in molecular techniques, it is now possible to measure astronomical (for a biologist, anyway) numbers of gene expression products simultaneously in single cells. Indeed, this approach is already offering promising results for the cataloguing of interneuronal species (Markram et al., 2004), albeit it is not yet entirely clear how the anatomically defined cell classes map onto the molecular classification schemes. A major limitation of the technique is that it detects mRNAs, not the actual proteins, nevertheless, the approach does have several advantages, highlighted by a series of recent studies.

Perhaps the most attractive feature of the approach lies in the possibility to arrive at a highly objective classification scheme for interneurons that can take into account a vast number of parameters simultaneously (as opposed to the candidate gene approach). Cauli et al. (2000) applied unsupervised cluster analysis to the classification of fusiform neocortical interneurons, based on multiple electrophysiological and molecular parameters obtained by patch clamp and single-cell multiplex reverse transcription-PCR (RT-PCR) techniques. Because this novel approach offers important insights that are likely to be relevant to our discussion here on diversity, we will consider this study in detail.

Three sets of parameters were considered by Cauli and colleagues (2000). The first set included 14 electrophysiological parameters (such as input resistence, first and second spike amplitude and duration and AHP, etc.). The second set of parameters considered nine interneuron-selective markers such as the general markers GAD65 and GAD67, as well as the more selectively expressed three calcium binding proteins (CB, PV, and CR), and four neuropeptides (NPY, VIP, SOM, and CCK). The last set included 25 parameters characterizing glutamate receptors (e.g., the AMPA receptor subunits GluR1-4, flip and flop variants, low-affinity kainate receptor subunits GluR5-7, high-affinity kainate receptor subunits KA1, KA2, the NMDA receptor subunits NR2A-D, and the metabotropic glutamate receptor subunits mGluR1-8). For the molecular data, the presence of a molecular product was considered as one, its absence as zero. To classify cells, Cauli et al. (2000) applied unsupervised clustering, where the analysis first groups the closest individuals (each of them being represented by a point in a multidimensional space, reminiscent of our discussion in chapter 4 about the various anatomical parameter axes for classification) by using the matrix of their Euclidean distances. At each stage, the number of groups is then decreased by at least one through the merging of those two groups or individuals whose combination leads to the smallest possible increase in the within-group sum of squared deviation. Importantly, the final number of clusters can be independently determined by a statistical process (known as the Thorndike procedure), which can determine the maximal decrease in the average within-cluster distance as the amalgamation procedure advances (Cauli et al., 2000).

Figure 7.5 illustrates their main results in the form of tree diagrams of cluster analysis applied to the sample of 85 neocortical neurons, based on either the expression of glutamate receptors (panel A1) or cellular markers (panel A2), or based on electrophysiological parameters (panel A3) or on different combinations of these parameters (panels B1–B3 and C). The first important conclusion was that only the combination of cellular markers and electrophysiological parameters (panel B3) allowed the segregation of pyramidal cells and fast spiking cells (which could be independently and reliably recognized) from the fusiform neurons. Application of the Thorndike procedure to the fusiform neurons clustered according to this latter combination of parameters resulted in three main groups of cells (actually, four groups, but branches 2b1 and 2b2 differed from each other only slightly and were later merged in a somewhat "supervised" manner): the regular spiking SOM^+ cells, the irregular spiking cells, and the regular spiking VIP^+ cells. Reassuringly, this separation of the heterogeneous fusiform group matches well with earlier studies.

Intriguingly, these results were achieved without considering morphological parameters. Perhaps the most important result was that the addition of glutamate receptors in the cluster analysis reduced the discriminative properties of the other parameters. Note that the consideration of all parameters (in panel C) resulted in a poorer segregation of the control pyramidal and fast spiking cells compared to the combination of the electrophysiological parameters and cellular markers, due the classification-blurring effects of the expression of glutamate receptors. In other words, the choice of parameters used in the cluster analysis was a critical decision for the determination of

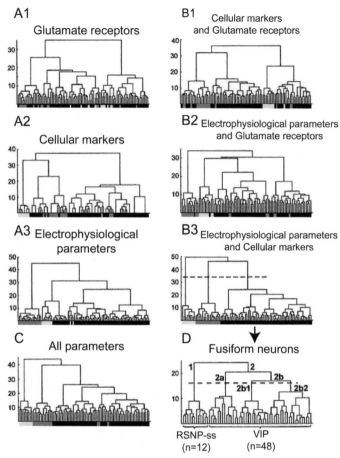

A1 Glutamate receptors

B1 Cellular markers and Glutamate receptors

A2 Cellular markers

B2 Electrophysiological parameters and Glutamate receptors

A3 Electrophysiological parameters

B3 Electrophysiological parameters and Cellular markers

C All parameters

D Fusiform neurons

RSNP-ss (n=12)   VIP (n=48)

Figure 7.5 **Comparison of different cluster analyses applied to neocortical fusiform interneurons** (black boxes, n = 60) as well as to pyramidal (white boxes, n = 9) and FS (gray boxes, n = 16) cells taken as controls. For each diagram, the x axis represents the individuals, and the y axis represents the average within-cluster linkage distance. Dotted lines in B3 and D indicate the limits between clusters as suggested by the Thorndike procedure. (A) Analyses based on the expression profiles of glutamate receptors (A1), of cellular markers (A2), or on electrophysiological properties (A3). (B and C) Analyses based on the combination of two of three sets of parameters (B1, B2, and B3) or on all parameters (C). Note that the control pyramidal and FS cells were segregated only by the combination of electrophysiological parameters and of cellular markers and that the expression of glutamate receptors blurs the classification. (D) Cluster analysis with the same parameters as in B3 restricted to the fusiform cell populaton. This analysis disclosed three groups of fusiform RSNP cells mainly expressing SS (RSNP-SS; branch labeled 1; n = 12) or mainly expressing VIP (branch labeled 2; n = 48). Within the group of VIP expressing cells, most of neurons of branch 2a were irregular spiking interneurons, and the majority of cells in branch 2b were RSNP cells. Within branch 2b, two subpopulations of RSNP-VIP (branches 2b1 and 2b2) were suggested by the Thorndike procedure. FS, fast spiking; RSNP, regular spiking nonpyramidal; SS, somatostatin; VIP, vasoactive intestinal polypeptide. Adapted, with permission, from Cauli et al. (2000).

neuronal subtypes. The actual reason for the latter result was that out of the 21 different glutamate receptors examined, only a few had cell-type specific expression. Thus, as the authors themselves concluded, the "definition of neuronal subtypes strongly depends on the discriminative properties of the criteria used. It is expected that electrophysiological or molecular parameters with low occurrence will have high discriminative potency." This surprising and important finding, that is, that the inclusion of a set of criteria (in this case, the expression of glutamate receptor subtypes) can actually reduce the discriminative properties of the other parameters, agrees well with our conclusions reached earlier in the second section of chapter 4, and it indicates that the classification may never be entirely unsupervised (i.e., the smart choice of a few marker genes outperforms the essentially "blind" consideration of vast numbers of parameters). Interestingly, similar conclusions regarding the degradation of cellular classification schemes by the blind addition of parameters have been reached also by recent studies in the retina (Kong et al., 2005).

Emerging Order in the Molecular Pandora's Box

Even though the molecular approach is not the panacea we may have hoped for, it does have a huge potential for future research into interneuronal diversity, especially because the essentially blind molecular dragnet approach can lead to the discovery of completely new, unexpected sets of genes that are expressed in a subtype-specific manner and whose protein products have not yet been considered in interneuronal research. We already touched upon the potential of the laser capture microdissection method in combination with microarray analysis for the issue of cellular heterogeneity (Kamme et al., 2003) in chapter 6. Cluster I in Fig 7.6 illustrates a cluster of genes that were highly expressed in one cell (cell number IX) but whose expression was much lower in the other cells (see also Fig. 6.9). Because one of these genes was parvalbumin, it was concluded that cell number IX was an interneuron (the others were most likely pyramidal cells). Two additional clusters of genes expressed in cell IX but not in the other cells were also identified (clusters II and III). Clearly, this analysis indicates that there are numerous genes that are potentially expressed in a highly subtype-specific manner. In order to verify that these candidate genes were indeed expressed in a selective

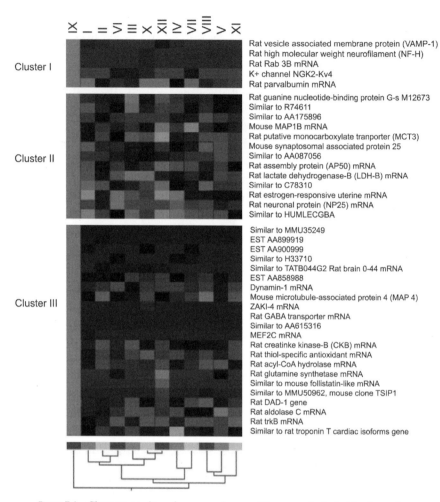

Figure 7.6 **Cluster tree view of expressed genes.** The genes included in three clusters are all expressed in cell IX but not expressed, or expressed at a lower level, in the remaining 11 cells. The column dendrogram at the bottom indicated that cell IX was dissimilar from the other cells. See also the related results in Fig. 6.9. Adapted, with permission, from Kamme et al. (2003).

fashion, five genes were selected for double in situ hybridization to validate the clustering results. The five selected genes were the GABA transporter-1 (GAT-1), neurofilament-H (NF-H), a K$^+$-channel subunit (NGK2-Kv4), the vesicle associated membrane protein 1 (VAMP1), and the myocyte enhancer factor-2C (MEF2C). The in situ results showed that, indeed, the expression of these genes was clearly colocalized with parvalbumin, and that NF-H and VAMP1 defined a subset of PV$^+$ cells. These results readily demonstrate the heuristic value of the molecular approach. For example, as already noted earlier, the expression of NF-H in parvalbumin-positive cells was described independently (Ratzliff & Soltesz, 2000), but that original discovery occurred only because the authors tested the somewhat unorthodox hypothesis that differential expression of neuronal cytoskeletal elements in interneurons may explain the curiously subtype-specific distribution of cellular damage after mechanical injury, delivered as a fast pressure-wave transient to the neocortex (Toth et al., 1997a). In other words, the unsupervised clustering approach has an immense potential for opening up the molecular Pandora's box for completely novel and entirely unexpected interneuron-specific gene expression patterns. If there are truly as many, perhaps hundreds and hundreds, of genes that are expressed in a cell type-specific manner as indicated by these studies (Kamme et al., 2003), it will be especially intriguing to see how many different interneuronal species could be differentiated based on the "one differentially expressed gene equals one interneuronal species" approach. Would we arrive at the grim prediction of the already discussed Parra et al. (1998) study, where each interneuron was a species to itself?

Only time will tell what the answer is to this daunting question. But efforts are already under way to apply cluster analysis of co-expression to interneurons (Markram et al., 2004; Toledo-Rodriguez et al., 2004). Perhaps most reassuringly, these studies revealed three main classes of ion-channel expression, which correlated surprisingly well with the expression of three calcium-binding proteins (PV, CB, and CR) that are already well-known as major marker proteins for the various interneuronal classes. The results thus revealed three major genes clusters. The "CR cluster" includes SK2, Kv3.4, and Caα1B (and, of course, CR itself). The "CB cluster" includes CB, Caβ4, HCN3m, Kv1.4m, Caα1G, Caβ1, HCN4, Kv3.3, and Caβ3. Finally, the third cluster, the "PV cluster", includes HCN2, Kv3.1, Kv1.2, Kv1.6, Kv1.1, PV, Kv3.2, HCN1, Kvβ1, and Caα1A (Markram et al., 2004). Importantly, as emphasized by Markram and his colleagues, the ion channels expressed in these three clusters might act in concert to generate three broad classes of discharge behavior. In general, ion channels in the CR cluster are associated with accommodation (Vergara et al., 1998), those in the CB cluster tend to promote bursting (Ertel et al., 1997), and those in the PV cluster tend to underlie high-frequency discharge (Martina et al., 1998; Chow et al.,

1999; Rudy & McBain, 2001). Thus, as pointed out above in connection with the Cauli et al. (2000) study, smart choice of marker genes, which have been (in a way, astonishingly presciently) identified and widely used by interneuronal anatomists during the past 20 years, have a bright future, especially in light of results that indicate the matching of the ion channel expressions with the expression patterns of the marker genes (Markram et al. 2004). In addition, the existence of such clusters indicate that perhaps there are only a handful of transcription factors that, expressed in different combinations, may regulate and determine the ultimate number and distinct properties of the interneuronal species. Clearly, the identification of these transcription factors will be crucial for understanding the nature of interneuronal species.

Ontogenetic Cladistics for Interneurons

The diversity of interneurons could be measured not only by species, but also by higher categories of classification. Biologists, for example, classify the domestic cat as follows: Species: *Felis domestica*; Genus: *Felis*; Family: Felidae; Order: Carnivora; Class: Mammalia; Phylum: Chordata; Kingdom: Animalia. A key principle of classification is the sharing of common ancestry (Wilson, 1992). For example, the species placed together in a genus are similar and share more or less immediate ancestry. Evidently, these classification schemes in biology refer to evolutionary ancestry, but, in our specific case regarding interneurons, the classification could also be applied to ontogenetic lineages. As discussed in chapter 2, it is clear that some interneuronal subtypes seem to be more closely related during development than others (e.g., parvalbumin-positive and somatostatin-positive interneurons originate from an embryonic area that seems to be distinct from the birthplace of the calretinin-containing interneurons). Thus, when more developmental data become available, ontogenetic trees may be constructed for interneurons at some point in the future, which could be used to devise higher-order classifications. The construction of branching patterns to map evolutionary change in biology is called cladistics. Ontogenetic cladistics, therefore, would reflect the successive splitting of interneuronal species through time during development (note that the devising of higher classifications could be correspondingly called ontogenetic systematics). Of course, the point here is that any higher-order classification for interneurons should be based on shared ontogenetic ancestry, which, in turn, needs detailed data on the origins of interneuronal species during ontogenesis. However, even before such data become available, work on classification may commence, based on our current anatomical, physiological, and immunocytochemical knowledge. Because parvalbumin expression, for example, seems to reflect the coexpression of a number of ion channel genes (see above), it is likely that the higher-order classifications designed purely on the basis of our current knowledge may turn out to be a pretty accurate reflection of the ontogenetic sharing of common ancestry. Therefore, parvalbumin-expressing interneuronal species (e.g., PV^+ basket and axo-axonic cells) would likely to be placed in the same interneuronal genus, whereas PV^+ interneurons and somatostatin-positive cells would also probably share a common, but perhaps even higher-order classification unit (e.g., family). But it is also clear that tough problems will be faced by researchers attempting to place interneurons into higher categories before the full developmental trees are constructed. For example, PV^+ and CCK^+ basket cells may be rather similar anatomically (e.g., in their postsynaptic target selectivity), but, as discussed earlier in chapter 3, they differ in a number of expressed receptors that endow them with distinct roles in the networks (Freund, 2003). Thus, there is no doubt that the ultimate answer regarding interneuronal systematics concerning higher-order categories will come from detailed fate-mapping and other developmental studies, which will be able to pinpoint, with increasing resolution, the common origins of the related interneuronal species.

Interneuronal Diversity and Evolution

Next, let's briefly consider the almost entirely unexplored area of interneuronal diversity and evolution. The widely accepted basic paradigm guiding interneuronal research is that each interneuronal species performs a set of specialized functions in the cortical networks, which, in turn, must have some, albeit perhaps currently not fully understood, behavioral consequences and relevance (e.g., Wang et al., 2004). Because many genes influence interneuronal species development (see chapter 2), it is likely that variation between the behavior of individual animals (or humans) is at least partly due to these genes. This issue is important, as evolution can only take place where variation in a feature is at least partly genetic, so that selection can act upon it. Let's consider the following argument by Slater and Halliday (1994):

> Genes, as such, do not cause behavioral patterns, and it is not necessary for them to do so for selection to affect behavior. To stress the point, all that is required is for variations in the behavior pattern to have some genetic component on which selection can act. It is hard to imagine any aspect of behavior of which this will not be true. Selection experiments may lead to change more or less quickly, depending on the extent to which individuals differ genetically in ways that affect the behavior, but it is hardly likely that such an experiment would not work at all. All behavior is genetically based, and affected by many genes; at least some of the variation in it is bound to stem from differences between individuals in their exact genotype.

Thus, if interneuronal species have specific functions in cortical networks, they are likely to influence behavior, and thus the genes that regulate the development of interneuronal subtypes (and other, nondevelopmental aspects of interneuronal properties) are likely to contribute to individual differences between members of an animal species. The branch of science that is concerned with the genetic analysis of individual differences in behavioral traits is behavioral genetics. How behavioral mutations alter the nervous system specifically falls under the scope of neurogenetics. In spite of successes in isolating genes and gene products involved in complex behaviors such as learning and memory (e.g., Dudai, 1988; Hoffmann, 1994), current neurogenetics has not yet put relevant evolutionary problems into the forefront. Although there are many studies looking at the genetic component of phenotypic variance (Hoffmann, 1994), it is unclear how variation specifically in those genes that affect interneuronal assembly and function in cortical networks underlie variation for traits relevant to an animal's ecology. However, many genes have been identified whose products are relevant to brain development, and some interesting results are already available in this regard. For example, the ASPM gene (the human orthologue of the *Drosophila melanogaster* abnormal spindle gene [asp], which is essential for normal mitotic spindle function in embryonic neuroblasts) is a key determinant of cerebral cortical size (Bond et al., 2002, 2003), through regulation of cell proliferation. Interestingly, there is evidence that the ASPM gene has been under strong selection in primates, and that the regions of the gene that are under selection in primates are the most highly diverged compared to other mammals (Evans et al., 2004; Kouprina et al., 2004). Therefore, these results provide evidence that genes that modulate cortical development can be under selection. Other cues may be gained from human neurogenetics that aims to determine the association of DNA polymorphism and human mental disorders through the study of the segregation of marker genes in affected and nonaffected families (e.g., Egeland et al., 1987), and, as we briefly discussed in chapter 2, some of these genes are likely to be involved in interneuronal development as well.

Although we are far from a full understanding of how genes modulating interneuronal species diversity play a role in phenotypic differences in ecologically relevant behavioral traits, there are recent, intriguing results that indicate that we may be able to start closing in on these questions. For example, a recent study showed how a polymorphism in the brain derived neurotrophic factor (BDNF) gene affects the anatomy of the hippocampus (Pezawas et al., 2004). A common val6met polymorphism in the BDNF gene affects intracellular packaging and regulated secretion of BDNF (Egan et al., 2003; Chen ct al., 2004) and also affects human hippocampal function and episodic memory (Egan et al., 2003; Hariri et al., 2003). Specifically, transfection of cultured hippocampal neurons with met-BDNF results in a reduction in depolarization-induced secretion and a failure to localize BDNF to secretary granules. Also, otherwise normal individuals that carry the met alleles have poorer episodic memory performance and reduced hippocampal engagement during memory studied with functional magnetic resonance imaging (fMRI) (Egan et al., 2003; Hariri et al., 2003). BDNF has been shown to modulate synaptic transmission and LTP (Figurov et al., 1996; Huang et al., 1999; Lee et al., 2004), and it also plays important roles in various developmental processes, including neuron survival, migration and differentiation, as well as activity-dependent modulation of synaptic structures (Huang et al., 1999; Gorski et al., 2003; Baquet et al., 2004; Hua & Smith, 2004). Based on these previous animal and human cognitive data, Pezawas and colleagues (2004) tested the hypothesis that met allele carriers had reduced hippocampal gray matter volume. In order to minimize environmental and ethnicity effects, only Caucasian subjects of European ancestry

were studied, who did not have any history of psychiatric or neurological illness, of psychiatric treatment, or of drug or alcohol abuse.
Out of the 111 subjects, 69 were val/val and 42 were met-carriers.
The fMRI data clearly demonstrated that the functional variation at
the val66met locus of the BDNF gene affected hippocampal morphology in humans, as the met-BDNF carriers had significantly
smaller hippocampal volume (on both sides; the decrease was about
15%). These differences were age and gender independent, suggesting that these changes occurred before adulthood. It is also noteworthy that BDNF is abundantly expressed throughout the human
brain, particularly in areas such as the prefrontal cortex implicated in
various psychiatric and neurological diseases. Indeed, further analysis showed that the met-BDNF carriers also exhibited reduced gray
matter volumes of extra-hippocampal loci including the prefrontal
cortex. Taken together, these data indicate that met-BDNF may lead
to stable alterations in cortical anatomy before adulthood, creating
an anatomical substrate related to variation in the function of distributed memory circuits (Egan et al., 2003). In support of this latter
suggestion, prefrontally targeted BDNF knockout mice displays similar decreases in cortical volume in adults (Baquet et al., 2004).

These human cortical data, therefore, take us a step closer to
the eventual unraveling of genetic variations that influence interneuronal networks. It is also worthwhile to note that many more
single-nucleotide polymorphisms are known, some of which are
associated with variation in cortical function. The best studied of
these is the polymorphism of catechol-O-methyltransferase (COMT),
which affects human executive cognition and physiology of the prefrontal cortex, most likely through modulation of dopamine signaling (COMT is an enzyme involved in the breakdown of dopamine)
(Egan et al., 2001; Akil et al., 2003), and the others include the
serotonin transporter promoter and a subtype of the metabotropic
glutamate receptor (Pezawas et al., 2004). Recent fMRI results concerning polymorphism of the human serotonin transporter gene
(SLC6A4) demonstrated allele-dependent neuronal network activity
(Heinz et al., 2005), where carriers of one particular allele (the so-
called short or s allele) displayed differential amygdala activity, and
greater amygdala to ventromedial prefrontal cortex coupling, upon
presentation of aversive, but not pleasant, pictures.

It is highly likely that at least some of these polymorphic genes
modulate interneuronal development and functions. For example,

BDNF strongly influences the development of several interneuronal subtypes, including, fast spiking interneurons (Berghuis et al., 2004). Although these are only the first steps in this exciting new field, it is clear that the question of how behaviorally relevant polymorphic genes alter interneuronal subtypes is an important one, which will need to be addressed in the future.

Constraints on Interneuronal Diversity

A class of questions that is closely related to the unsolved problems outlined in the previous section concerns the issue of ontogenetic and evolutionary constraints on interneuronal species diversity. Developmental processes may play a key role in keeping the intragroup, cell-to-cell variance at a level that is low enough to allow the emergence and persistence of interneuronal species, but the nature of these regulatory forces is not yet understood. Ontogenetic constraints may also place an upper limit on how many distinct interneuronal species may exist, perhaps because only so many different cell classes may emerge from any one embryonic area such as the medial ganglionic eminence at any one time, possibly due to limitations on the steepness of concentration gradients for diffusible regulatory molecules or to some other factor. It is also possible that early prenatal development is only responsible for the creation of broad interneuronal classes (e.g., families, as discussed earlier in this chapter in relation to ontogenetic cladistics), and it is the later, possibly including the postnatal environmental, factors that further chisel out the finer interneuronal subgroups. From the point of view of evolutionary constraints, it is also interesting to wonder how selection may act on individual differences to guide the emergence of the various, distinct interneuronal species that we encounter today in cortical networks. The truth is that we just do not know the answers to these puzzles. But these questions are fascinating and important, and it is likely that an increasing number of interneuronal researchers will start focusing on these questions. For example, it has been known since the early 1960s (Broadhurst, 1960) that distinct lines can be created in rats and mice by selecting over successive generations for individual animals with low and high emotionality scores (measured as the rate of urination or defecation when placed in a new environment), indicating that genetic differences existed between individuals, and that these behavioral traits (similar to morphological or physiological traits) can be subjected to genetic analysis (Hoffman, 1994). In spite of the availability of such data for many decades, we still do not know whether specific interneuronal species differ between such lines of rats or mice. Of course, the main reason for this delay has been that the various interneuronal species needed to be first defined and agreed upon. With the revolution in interneuronal research in the 1990s due to the emergence of a constellation of new technical possibilities, such as patch clamp recordings and molecular analysis of large numbers of genes, these questions can be addressed in the near future.

An insightful attempt at calculating the upper limit on cortical interneuronal types came from the application of the so-called "tiling principle," originally described in the retina, to the neocortex and hippocampus by Stevens (1998). The tiling principle of the retina originated from the initial observations by Wassle and colleagues (1981) that some ganglion cell types just cover the retina with their dendritic fields. The generality of this rule was demonstrate later by DeVries and Baylor (1997), who showed that the receptive fields of any particular type of neighboring ganglion cell overlap only insignificantly, but every part of the retina is well covered by a receptive field of that cell type. Thus, every locality in the retina, and thus in the visual field, is covered by the dendrites of any particular ganglion cell type. Now let's imagine that this tiling principle applies to other brain areas, and see what happens if we calculate the upper limit of interneuronal species in the hippocampus. Here is Stevens' argument (Stevens, 1998):

> Underneath 1 mm^2 of hippocampal cortex in the CA1 region, one finds about 5×10^4 neurons, perhaps 10% or 20% of which are inhibitory. If we take the fraction of inhibitory neurons to be 0.1, then our standard piece of cortex will contain something like 5×10^3 inhibitory neurons. Suppose that each of these has a dendritic field that is 300 µm in diameter, so that, looking down on the cortical surface, its dendrites could cover an area of about 0.07 mm^2. It would take 14 neurons like this to cover our standard 1 mm^2 of cortex, and so there could be up to 350 types of inhibitory neurons because the available inhibitory neurons could tile the cortical surface 350 times over.

Of course, one can raise doubt about the applicability of the tiling principle to the cortex. However, it seems reasonable to assume that no part of a cortical network, such as the hippocampus, lacks a particular kind of interneuron, if that interneuron is truly important for the computations. Thus, in this light, the application of the tiling argument to the cortex may not be so far-fetched. The above-quoted argument, indicating that there could be at least as many as 350 types of interneuronal species, is a lot more than the number of interneuronal classes that we are currently aware of (e.g., see Fig. 3.1). But the number of 350 types may not be completely out of the plausible range either, especially if we consider that recent studies using high-throughput, innovative anatomical techniques identified no less than 22 distinct morphological types just within the class of amacrine cells (MacNeil & Masland, 1998; Masland, 2001). Extension of the tiling argument to the primate neocortex yielded an even more frightening estimate than in the hippocampus, something in the order of about 600 types (Stevens, 1998). In the end, of course, "arm-chair arguments" such as these can only guess the outer limits of interneuronal diversity, and it will be only through painstaking identification of individual species that we can assemble the tree of interneuronal life.

8

Fifty Ways to Be a Basket Cell: Self-Tuning Interneurons with Multiple Solutions for Their Tasks

----

> *... individual neurons of the same class may each have found an acceptable solution to a genetically determined pattern of activity ....*
>
> Eve Marder and Astrid Prinz (2002)

The "Ideal" Basket Cell

In chapter 1, we introduced the problem of idealization of cell types, in connection with Mayr's warning. We can now return to this issue to examine it in a new light, aided by the preceding discussions in chapters 3–7 on interneuronal heterogeneity. A good starting point is to remind ourselves of the main problem, presented as two mutually exclusive alternatives: Is the neuronal machine built from rigidly predetermined, precisely manufactured, identical individuals of interneuronal species that are being inserted into the machine to perform a set of highly specialized functions? Or, are interneuronal species more like distinct distributions of forms and molecular properties, where each interneuronal species forms a population with certain cell-to-cell variability, with the variability being just important for its functions at the network level? As evident from the preceding chapters, we believe that the answer is yes to the latter question. But is it even biologically realistic to believe that the basket cells are manufactured with great precision to have the exact, right combinations of ion channels to produce a predetermined output? What would the ideal (say) PV^+ basket cell look like? Is there only a single combination of ion channel expression that would allow the PV^+ basket cells to fulfill their functional roles in the network?

As discussed in chapter 7, certain ion channels, such as Kv3.1, are associated with the typically fast spiking PV$^+$ cells (Martina et al., 1998; Rudy & McBain, 2001), and clusters of gene expression appear to underlie and govern the "forward engineering" of electrical behavior for the various interneuronal types (Markram et al., 2004). Thus, in this sense, we may talk about a "typical" or "ideal" PV$^+$ basket cell. But does that mean that the network is made up of essentially identical PV$^+$ basket cells, where the cell-to-cell difference is purely due to experimental measurement errors or perhaps to some inherent limitation of the biological system, which tries to approximate the "ideal" as much as possible, but is limited by imperfect tools or by some unavoidable noise?

Could there be some deeper reason why two PV$^+$ basket cells (or any two cells belonging to the same subtype) are never identical? Is the "typical" form just a fiction of our imagination? It is useful to remind ourselves how we usually build such typified representations of interneuronal species, namely, by measuring the intrinsic or synaptic conductances in a (preferably) large number of PV$^+$ basket cells over many months and years, from many animals, often in several laboratories, on different strains or even species, and then we average these measurements to arrive at the mean, the "typical" basket cell. But is this procedure necessarily correct?

In this chapter, we will show how multiple "solutions" to a particular cell type's function in a network may exist in the form of numerous, equally functional combination of conductances. Furthermore, we will also discuss evidence that indicates that the "mean cell" created from individuals belonging to a particular cell type may not even function like the cell type from which it was created. Finally, we will discuss an alternative paradigm, where it is the target activity levels that are tightly controlled, and not the number of each kind of ion channel individually.

Unbearable Multiplicity of Being a Specialized Neuron

In order to determine whether a basket cell needs tightly predetermined levels of expression for each conductance to perform its functions, the ideal experiment would be to record ion channel conductances from the same individual basket cell over the course of days, under similar behavioral conditions. This dream experiment is, of course, not yet possible. But something akin to this dream experiment can be achieved in the simpler (or, at least smaller) nervous system of the crab *Cancer borealis*, where each class of identified neurons in the somatogastric ganglion displays a characteristic and stereotyped firing pattern. In this nervous system, one can identify a particular cell, which presumably has a set of computational tasks to perform for the benefit of the animal, as indicated by the stereotyped firing pattern.

Because the same neuron can be identified in different individual crabs, one can address the question of whether that particular cell in the network with the given functional task expresses identical sets of ion channel conductances. When this experiment was performed on one particular cell in the network, the inferior cardiac neuron, the results showed something truly astonishing (Golowasch et al., 2002). In spite of the stereotyped behavior, when peak conductances were measured in 22 different preparations in the inferior cardiac neuron, the results revealed a very large amount of variability in the measured peak values for 3 K^+-conductances (Fig. 8.1). Specifically, there was a three- to fourfold (!) variation between the maximal conductance values for the A-type, delayed rectifier-, and the Ca^{2+}-activated K^+-conductances.

The observed variability was certainly beyond what most of us would expect to see in cell-to-cell differences within a single neuronal subtype, if the differences were solely due to experimental error or to some inherent limitation of the system. These data from Golowasch and colleagues (2002) suggest that there are many possible combinations of ion channel conductance values that allow individual cells belonging to precisely the same neuronal subtype to properly function in the network of the somatogastric ganglion of different individual animals.

Failure of Averaging

How is it possible to have such large variations in peak conductances, and still function as an inferior cardiac neuron? To answer this question, a model neuron was built by Golowasch and colleagues with 5 voltage-dependent conductances, and 2,000 variants of this model neuron were produced by randomly choosing sets of maximal conductances (Golowasch et al., 2002). The resulting model neurons

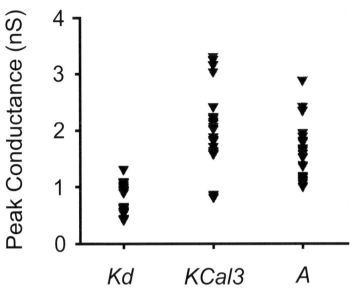

Figure 8.1 **Variation in the peak conductances of three K$^+$ conductances for a neuron of the crab stomatogastric ganglion (STG).** Peak conductances measured in the inferior cardiac (IC) neuron of 22 different preparations vary over a factor of 3.1 for gKd, 4.0 for gKCa, and 2.9 for gA. Means and SDs for the three conductances are as follows: gKd = 0.77 ± 0.27 nS, gKCa = 6.05 ± 2.15 nS, gA = 1.58 ± 0.50 nS. Reprinted, with permission, from Golowasch et al. (2002).

were classified as silent, tonically firing or bursting with a certain number of spikes per burst. Out of the 2,000 model cell variants, 164 were identified as "one-spike bursting neurons" (Fig. 8.2). A major finding was that, as shown on the right in Fig. 8.2A, the same firing pattern (one-spike bursting) could be generated by a large variety of Na$^+$- and Kd-conductances. In the case of the top cell (cell no. 1), for example, the one-spike bursting was achieved with a lot of Na$^+$-conductance but little Kd, opposite to cell no. 3, which was also a one-spike burster, but had small g_{max}Na and high g_{max}Kd.

And here comes an even more surprising, key finding. Even though there were many "solutions" to the problem of being a one-spike burster, the average of these solutions did not result in a one-spike burster model neuron (Fig. 8.2B)! Specifically, when the mean g_{max}Na and g_{max}Kd was calculated from the 164 one-spike bursters, the resulting cell was a three-spike burster neuron, clearly different from the defining property of the 164 cells that led to its creation through averaging. This important result, therefore, represents the

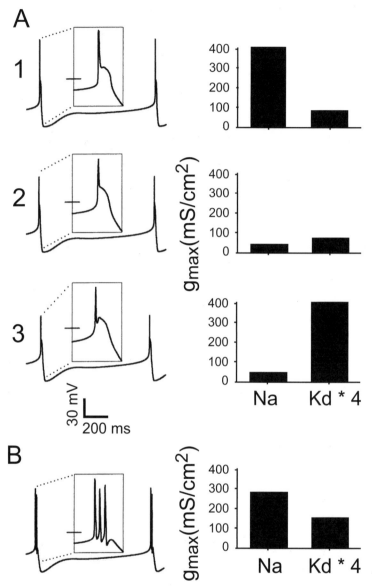

Figure 8.2 **Failure of averaging in a conductance-based model neuron.** (A) Left panels: voltage traces for three observed one-spike bursters. Conductance values in mS/cm2: 1, $g_{max}Na = 400$, $g_{max}Kd = 20.0$; 2, $g_{max}Na = 50.0$, $g_{max}Kd = 20.0$; 3, $g_{max}Na = 50.0$, $g_{max}Kd = 100$; all three, $g_{max}Ca = 4.0$, $g_{max}A = 5.0$, $g_{max}KCa = 250$. (B) Neuron generated from the average conductances of all the one-spike bursters ($g_{max}Na = 283$, $g_{max}Kd = 38.0$, $g_{max}Ca = 3.45$, $g_{max}A = 26.2$, $g_{max}KCa = 146$). The insets are 50 ms in width and have tick marks at –30 mV. Right panels: histograms showing the values of the Na^+ and four times the delayed-rectifier K^+ maximal conductances. Reprinted, with permission, from Golowasch et al. (2002).

failure of averaging as a means of creating a "typical" or idealized neuron of a certain type. The implication for this finding is enormous for interneuron research, as it is precisely through the creation of such averages that we build our single cell (conceptual or computational) models. It is also important to emphasize that the underlying reason for the failure of averaging is that, in complex model neurons with a number of distinct conductances, similar firing properties can be produced by widely different combinations of conductances (as also evident in Fig. 8.2A), and the phenotype depends not on one single conductance, but on the correlated levels of several conductances. A significant consequence of this fact is that the effect of changing the number of channels of one current may strongly differ, depending on the numbers of each of the other kinds of channels in that particular neuron. It should be also noted that the averaged neuron *can* be, in certain cases, similar to the individual, pooled neurons, but not necessarily so, as the data in Fig. 8.2 illustrate.

Figure 8.3 explains why averaging fails in this particular case. Each dot in Fig. 8.3A represents one out of the 2,000 combinations of g_{max}Na and g_{max}Kd used in the above-discussed model (Golowasch et al., 2002). As can be seen in the figure, the one-spike bursters lie in an L-shaped region, because they are defined by low values of g_{max}Na and/or g_{max}Kd. The mean, and most of the points within the ellipse delineating 1 SD of the mean, fall outside of this region that defined the one-spike bursters. Thus, the mean of the one-spike bursters is not a one-spike burster cell. The figure also shows that for multiple bursters, which are scattered fairly evenly in the plot, the mean value would likely give a multiple burster (although the mean of, say, three-spike bursters may not necessarily result in a three-spike bursting neuron).

Homeostatic Regulation and Activity Sensors

A key assumption of the mean-based approach, where pooled data are used to create an idealized cell of a certain kind, is that all of the individual neurons have essentially the same set of conductances, and that any measured differences in conductance densities between individual cells are produced by experimental (measurement) errors. But, as seen in the previous section, perhaps this assumption

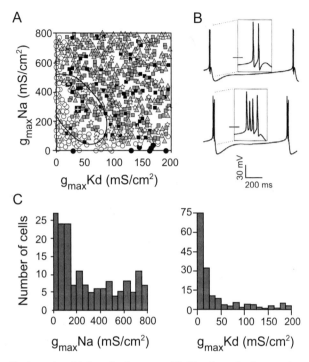

Figure 8.3 **Single and multiple spike bursters.** (A) Number of spikes per burst (0, black circle; 1, white circle; 2, gray triangle; 3, gray square; 4, black square; 5, white star) for bursting neurons with the indicated values of $g_{max}Na$ and $g_{max}Kd$. One-spike bursters (white circle) lie in an L-shaped region that *does not include its mean* (black square with cross, which generates the activity seen in panel B in the previous figure) or most of its 1 SD covariance ellipse (black oval curve; individual conductance SDs in mS/cm2 are $_{Na} = 241$; $_{Kd} = 50.6$; $_{Ca} = 1.18$; $_{A} = 20.1$; $_{KCa} = 88.6$). Bursters with more than 1 spike per burst appear randomly distributed in this two-dimensional projection. (B) Voltage traces for two neurons (a two-spike burster and a four-spike burster) with conductances lying within 1 SD of the mean (conductance values in mS/cm²: upper trace, $g_{max}Na = 229$, $g_{max}Kd = 60.2$, $g_{max}Ca = 2.72$, $g_{max}A = 36.0$, $g_{max}KCa = 158$; lower trace, $g_{max}Na = 296$, $g_{max}Kd = 26.4$, $g_{max}Ca = 2.89$, $g_{max}A = 15.5$, $g_{max}KCa = 90.6$). The insets are 50 ms in width and have tick marks at –30 mV. (C) Distribution histograms showing the number of one-spike bursting neurons with the indicated amount of $g_{max}Na$ (left) or $g_{max}Kd$ (right). Adapted, with permission, from Golowasch et al. (2002).

may not be entirely valid, as the same kind of behavior can be produced by different sets of conductances. Instead of tightly regulating the density of each and every conductance in every single cell belonging to a certain cell type, it may be much simpler and more effective to have a mechanism that adjusts the conductances according to a target activity level.

The basic idea that neurons can self-tune to find a combination of conductance densities consistent with a target activity level and pattern was tested in a number of models (Marder & Prinz, 2002). The premise was that intracellular sensors can detect activity levels drifting away from the equilibrium state, and these sensors trigger alterations in the number and/or distribution of conductances. Because intracellular Ca^{2+}-levels were shown to fluctuate according to activity (Ross, 1989; Bito et al., 1997), intracellular Ca^{2+}-sensors seemed ideal for the purpose of sensing activity levels and triggering changes in conductance levels (Abbott & LeMasson, 1993; LeMasson et al., 1993). If activity decreases, the intracellular Ca^{2+}-concentration falls below he target level, triggering increases in depolarizing membrane currents and downregulation of hyperpolarizing membrane currents, and vice versa. It should be noted that the midpoint for the Ca^{2+}-sensor and the regulation time constant could be different for different conductances, and that multiple Ca^{2+}-sensors working on different timescales make it possible to change conductance densities much slower than the timescales involved in neuronal signaling.

An illuminating example is shown in Fig. 8.4. The model has two Ca^{2+} currents, a Na^{+}-current, three K^{+}-currents, and three activity sensors. The figure shows the maximal conductances changing with time, with example voltage traces at the indicated points. Note that, as the neuron approached its equilibrium state, it decreased in Na^{+}-conductance and also changed all its other conductances. Again, as we have already seen in the previous section, similar activity patterns could be produced at several points along the adjustment process (e.g. 3, 5, 6, 7, 8). As the neuron converged to its equilibrium point, large changes in conductances could occur with relatively little alterations in firing properties.

These simulation results with self-tuning of conductances to produce target activity levels in a homeostatic manner were closely supported by experiments on cultured neurons. These now-classical experiments by Turrigiano and colleagues (Turrigiano et al., 1994; Desai et al., 1999) showed that when activity levels were suppressed in cultured neurons for days with the Na^{+}-channel blocker tetrodotoxin (TTX), the neurons turned out to be more excitable (following the washout of TTX). The increased excitability, furthermore, was shown to be due to an upregulation of Na^{+}-conductances and downregulation of K^{+}-conductance densities. It should also be mentioned here

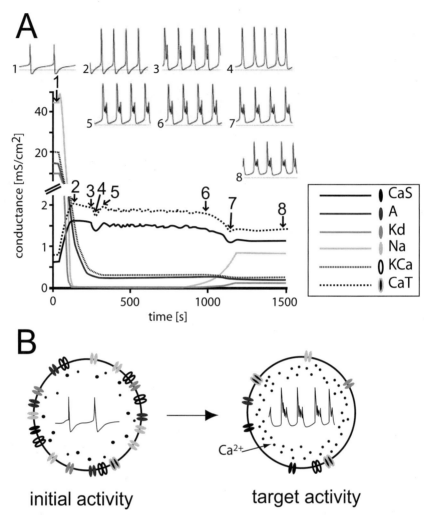

Figure 8.4 **Activity-dependent conductance regulation in a model neuron with three calcium sensors.** (A) Maximal conductances (the traces corresponding to the various conductances were coded as indicated on the lower right) and voltage traces at different times (insets) as a regulating model neuron approaches its target activity. Note that similar firing patters (3, 5–8) result from different combinations of conductances during the regulation process. (B) Cartoon illustrating the downregulation of the sodium, calcium-dependent and transient potassium, and delayed rectifier conductances and upregulation of the transient and slow calcium conductances (symbols corresponding to the various conductances are coded as indicated in panel A on the lower right) between the initial state of the model and its target activity and the accompanying increase in intracellular calcium to the target level. Adapted, with permission, from Marder and Prinz (2002).

that, in addition to conductance densities or distributions, tuning could also take place through changes in the voltage dependency of currents, and homeostatic regulation could also occur with synaptic conductances. When activity levels are suppressed or elevated, inhibitory inputs decrease or increase, respectively, and the excitatory synaptic conductances also follow this general homeostatic principle (Turrigiano et al., 1998; Turrigiano & Nelson, 2000; Watt et al., 2000; Leslie et al., 2001; Kilman et al., 2002). An interesting aspect of these findings was that they indicated that neurons can regulate their total synaptic drive, that is, the strength of all of their synaptic inputs, through a mechanism that was named "synaptic scaling" (Turrigiano et al., 1998). The basic homeostatic principle was shown to work at *Drosophila* neuromuscular junctions (here the activity levels were decreased in a prolonged manner by the overexpression of K-channels) (Davis & Bezprozvanny, 2001; Paradis et al., 2001), as well as at the *Xenopus* neuromuscular junction (Nick & Ribera, 2000).

Homeostasis in GABAergic Systems

Obviously, much more will be needed to be learnt about homeostatic mechanisms in the future. For example, the bulk of the biological data regarding homeostatic regulation is from cultured neurons and not from in vivo situations. Furthermore, little attention has been paid in the past to how cell-wide homeostatic mechanisms may affect GABAergic conductances underlying the various interneuronal inputs. But there are interesting, novel modeling results concerning the tuning of GABAergic conductances (Soto-Trevino et al., 2001) in a three-cell network of the crustacean pyloric rhythm. Two rules were implemented in these studies for the tuning of synaptic conductances. One was global, which took into account the neuron's total excitability, akin to synaptic scaling. The other rule was local, synapse specific, which was concerned with the effectiveness of each presynaptic neuron in influencing the activity of the postsynaptic cell. Starting with randomly assigned synaptic strength, these two rules allow the network to assemble into a functional, rhythmic circuit. In a manner that is reminiscent of the multiple solutions to a single cell type discussed above, the networks during the tuning process found many parameter regions over which almost identical network dynamics could be observed (Soto-Trevino et al., 2001). Thus, it may not be necessary to perfectly tune each synapse in order to arrive at acceptable physiological outputs, just like it may not be necessary to perfectly tune each and every conductance in a neuron to arrive at an acceptable firing pattern output (Marder & Prinz, 2002; Prinz, et al., 2004; Bucher, et al., 2005).

Homeostatic regulation may also take place at long timescales at individual perisomatic GABAergic synapses (Santhakumar & Soltesz, 2004). Seizures and trauma taking place in vivo are particularly useful in gaining insights into long-term plasticity mechanisms in GABAergic systems, including their relationships to homeostatic plasticity mechanisms (Mody, 2005). Seizures and trauma have been reported to lead to long-term alterations in GABA release (Chen et al., 1999; Hirsch et al., 1999), changes in the number and subunit composition of $GABA_A$ receptors (Houser & Esclapez, 2003), retraction of GABAergic dendrites (Nitsch & Frotscher, 1992), sprouting of axons (Arellano et al., 2004), changes in resting membrane potential (Ross & Soltesz, 2000), excitatory synaptic drive (Doherty & Dingledine, 2001; Santhakumar et al., 2001), and rhythmicity and synchrony of sIPSC bursts (Chen et al., 2001). Albeit the many variants of synaptic and cellular alterations is daunting, it has been suggested that the diverse, seemingly disparate alterations in various interneuronal parameters frequently observed in animal models of human neurological conditions may be tied together by homeostatic mechanisms (Santhakumar & Soltesz, 2004). It is especially interesting to consider the plasticity mechanisms at hippocampal perisomatic GABAergic synapses after fever-induced (febrile) seizures. These developmental seizures lead to three distinct, functionally opposing alterations involving both pre- and postsynaptic sites, including the presynaptic enhancement of perisomatic GABAergic transmission (Chen et al., 1999), the postsynaptic upregulation of the hyperpolarization activated cation current (I_h) (Chen et al., 2001), and an augmentation in the number of presynaptic cannabinoid type 1 (CB1) receptors (Chen et al., 2003). The potentiated GABA release is counteracted by the increased I_h that limits the inhibitory postsynaptic potentials (IPSPs) (Chen et al., 2001), and by the elevated number of CB1 receptors that strongly depresses GABA release through a process known as depolarization-induced suppression of inhibition (Chen et al., 2003). These results suggest that homeostatic mechanisms may underlie several, seemingly disparate synaptic and cellular changes in GABAergic systems in neurological diseases (Turrigiano & Nelson, 2004), and they are in general agreement with the recent data from both *in vitro* and *in vivo* studies discussed above, indicating that homeostatic processes can powerfully regulate both excitatory and inhibitory synaptic transmission as well as intrinsic excitability. It should be mentioned here that the apparent involvement of homeostatic processes does not necessarily mean that the post-insult network fully regained its original functional properties (Santhakumar & Soltesz, 2004). Some homeostatic processes may be maladaptive, and actually contribute to the pathological state. For example, the enhanced I_h after the seizures may oppose the increased GABA-release in a homeostatic sense, but it can also result in the appearance of novel properties, such as postinhibitory rebound firing after the arrival of a barrage of IPSPs, that would be expected to contribute to hyperexcitability (Chen et al., 2001.

Wanted, Alive: Interneuronal Heterogeneity in Naturalistic Environments

In this chapter, we hope that a compelling case was presented for the biological necessity of having multiple solutions for the computational tasks of being a specialized interneuron. It seems that it is much more biologically plausible to have each interneuron self-tune its conductances to achieve an acceptable, physiologically relevant output through the automatic, activity-dependent self-tuning of its conductances rather than rigidly predetermining the exclusively "correct" amount of each of the numerous conductances that an interneuron expresses. In a similar way, it seems also plausible that the same dynamic behavior may be attained through the cell-wide self-tuning of synapses, freeing the system from the rather daunting requirement of individually determining and regulating every single conductance and synapse. In terms of its simplicity, there is no doubt that it makes more sense to imagine multiple solutions and many possible and actual implementations to the task of being, say, a basket cell, as opposed to trying to get as close as possible to the idealized, average basket cell, especially because that "average" basket cell may turn out to be not a basket cell after all (see above). Thus, taken together, the experimental and modeling results from the

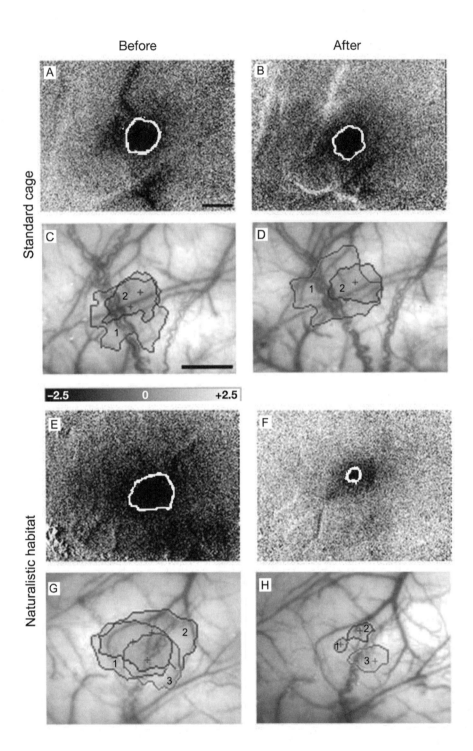

Before After

Standard cage

−2.5 0 +2.5

Naturalistic habitat

168

laboratories from Eve Marder, Larry Abbott, Gina Turrigiano, Sacha Nelson, and others indicate that there is a deep biological reason why cell-to-cell variability exists in real networks, even within well-defined interneuronal populations.

Before we close this chapter, let's return to one more important problem. We mentioned in the above section that there is a paucity of in vivo data on homeostatic mechanisms, especially when it comes to GABAergic processes. However, there is another aspect to this issue, namely, that there is a difference between in vivo as an animal in a standard cage versus in vivo where the animal behaves in a naturalistic environment. In chapter 6, we briefly touched upon the question of how environmental influences may modulate interneuronal cell-to-cell variability. Because we believe that this issue is a potentially crucially important subject for interneuronal heterogeneity as well as to the question of homeostatic regulation of GABAergic systems, we revisit this question here briefly.

It has been known for some time that sensory deprivation during development can cause substantial changes in GABAergic cells and synapses. For example, after whisker removal in the early postnatal rat, there is a permanent, dramatic decrease in the number of GABAergic synapses (particularly those on dendritic spines in the thalamo-recipient layer IV) and cells in the necortex (Micheva & Beaulieu, 1997). Although these and similar sensory deprivation studies in rodents and other species (e.g., Jones, 1993, 2002) are important and interesting, they raise some additional questions. For example, when a whisker is functionally removed, the control rat is supposed to be a normal rat that uses its whiskers in a natural fashion. But is that really true? Is the typical control rat that is sitting in

Figure 8.5 **Chronic optical imaging of functional whisker representations through the intact skull.** For all panels, boundaries demarcate cortical areas with intrinsic signal activity 2.5×10^{-4}. (A, B, E, F) Ratio images of the C2 whisker representation collected before (A and E) and after (B and F) exposure to standard cage (SC) (A and B) or naturalistic habitat (NH) (E and F). Grayscale bar indicates intrinsic signal strength $\times 10^{-4}$. Black and white streaks correspond to large surface blood vessels. Scale bar in (A), which also applies to (B), (E), and (F), = 1 mm. (C, D, G, H) Functional representations for whisker C1 (area labeled "2"), C2 (area labeled "1"), and B2 (area labeled "3"; in G and H) obtained from two different SC (C and D) and NH (G and H) rats, superimposed onto images of the cortical surface as seen through the thinned skull before (C and G) and after (D and H) exposure. Functional peaks for each whisker are indicated by a cross. Scale bar in (C), which also applies to (D), (G), and (H), = 1 mm. Adapted, with permission, from Polley et al. (2004).

its cage all day a truly normal animal? Or are the rat's whiskers destined to be used to be heavily stimulated during burrowing through ground and debris, in a constantly changing and complex tactile and spatial environment, which would not occur, or would not occur to the same degree, in a rat sitting in its laboratory cage? These questions are crucial, as most of what we know about cortical microcircuits arose from observations made in rodents kept in standard laboratory cages.

A recent, elegant study (Polley et al., 2004) addressed this issue in an especially illuminating manner. Polley and colleagues showed that placing rats from their standard cages into a naturalistic habitat dramatically transformed both the morphological and functional facial whisker representation in the somatosensory cortex. Although the authors did not specifically address the question of interneuronal involvement in this plasticity, it is highly likely that interneurons were affected by such large-scale refinement of cortical sensory maps, especially considering the fact the whisker ("barrel") representations shrank by almost half(!) after the exposure to the environment that allowed the expression of the animals' innate behaviors such as digging, burrowing, and subterranean tunneling (Fig. 8.5). Importantly, these rats were adult rats, therefore, these observations are distinct from the well-known plasticity of cortical whisker representation in the barrel cortex, which is strictly limited to the first week of postnatal life (Van der Loos & Woolsey, 1973; Jeanmonod et al., 1981). Based on the laminar specificity of these changes (layers II/III were especially affected), the authors suggested that alterations in intracortical circuits may have underlied these effects. It is interesting to note from this respect that studies have shown that, after 24 hours of whisker stimulation, there is a long-lasting increase in GABAergic synaptic inputs to spines, indicating that enhanced activity of whiskers can lead to plasticity of interneuronal processes lasting for days (Knott et al., 2002). Because, as mentioned above, the overwhelming majority of our knowledge on interneuronal species comes from studies conducted on rats and mice housed in standard laboratory cages, future investigations will need to address how intraspecies variability and species diversity in interneuronal networks are altered by exposure to naturalistic environments. These much-needed studies will also certainly help to determine how homeostatic mechanisms regulate interneuronal processes in a genuinely freely moving animal.

9

Interneuronal Diversity and Small-World Neuronal Networks

This is the remarkable paradox of mathematics: no matter how determinedly its practitioners ignore the world, they consistently produce the best tools for understanding it.

J. Tierney (1984)

Building Complex Machines with Minimal Wiring

As mentioned earlier in chapter 1, Cajal, based on his observations from Golgi material obtained from various animal species, had already suggested that interneuronal diversity may be higher in animals with higher intelligence (e.g., in humans compared to rodents). Whether Cajal's suggestion is true or not is still an open question. For example, it is not entirely clear if there are more interneuronal species in the human compared to the rat hippocampus, and the relative abundance of the interneuronal species is also not known (note that both the total number of species and their relative abundance would be needed to give a quantitative answer to the issue of evolutionary changes in interneuronal diversity). But it is clear that evolution needed to solve the basic problem of ever-increasing demand on neuronal network performance. In general, there are two classes of solutions for the problem of enhancing network performance (Buzsáki et al., 2004). First, one can use a large number of few constituents. This simple approach, however, soon runs into a problem, simply because of physical size. As the network grows, space and energy limitations will become more and more severe. The second approach is to increase network performance by adding novel types of constituents (i.e., increasing the number of interneuronal species). The addition of new elements should enable the networks to carry out new computations; for example, oscillations at new frequencies (Buzsáki et al., 2004). This second solution, proposing to increase network performance by increasing the diversity of computational elements, is clearly less constrained by physical and energy-related problems.

But how did evolution hook up networks with diverse computing elements? Or, to ask the same question in another way, what is the basic architectural design of neuronal networks? A recent insight into this interesting question came from an entirely unexpected source, namely, from studies that applied graph theoretical techniques to real-world networks ranging from the biochemical and social networks to the electrical grid of the United States and the Internet (Watts & Strogatz, 1998; Barabási & Albert, 1999; Albert et al., 2000; Jeong et al., 2000). In a landmark paper, Watts and Strogatz (1998) contrasted two types of networks, the highly ordered, regular networks, and random networks (Fig. 9.1). They employed two measures, the average shortest path length (L, the average number of steps one has to take to go from any "node" to any other node on average) and the clustering coefficient (C, describing the probability that two nodes connected to a common node are also connected to each other) to characterize network architecture. It is easy to get an intuitive feel for these measures. In human societies, for example, L can describe how many people (or "handshakes") separate any of us from each other on this planet. Its popularized version is the famous "six degrees of separation" between any individual and (for example) the president of the United States (I know someone who knows someone … who knows the president) (Milgram, 1967; Guare, 1990). The clustering coefficient C, again in human terms, describes the probability that my friends know each other (because human societies tend to be "cliquish," C is typically high). In highly ordered networks (Fig. 9.1, left panel), individual nodes are richly linked to their neighbors (high C), but it takes a lot of steps to go from a node to other nodes on average (high L). In random networks containing the same number of nodes and links (Fig. 9.1, right panel), the L is low, but the local connectivity is relatively poor (low C). Watts and Strogatz's main insight was that, if even a few links from the ordered network are reconnected in a random fashion, the resulting network will be unlike any of these other two networks, because they will have a low L (like random networks, due to the presence of long-range connections) and a high C (like regular net-

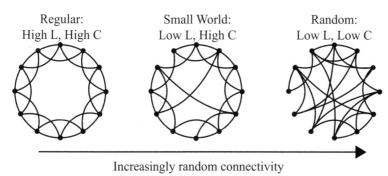

Figure 9.1 **Small-world networks.** Basic types of graph structure (regular, small-world, and random) are illustrated, with the characteristic L and C values indicated above the graphs. Based on Watts and Strogatz (1998). Reprinted, with permission, from Földy et al. (2005).

works). They called these types of networks between ordered and random networks "small-world" networks.

As mentioned above, there are many, diverse examples of real life technical, biological, and social ("six degrees of separation") networks that are small-world networks (Watts & Strogatz, 1998; Albert et al., 1999; Barabási et al., 2000; Jeong et al., 2000). The key property of these small-world networks is that a few randomly placed shortcuts (i.e., long-distance links) can dramatically reduce the L of ordered networks, with the local connectivity remaining high (Watts, 1999; Barabási, 2002; Buchanan, 2002;). Computational models have shown that such networks have several advantages for neuronal networks. One of the earliest modeling results on the subject came from a paper in *Physical Review Letters* by Lago-Fernandez and colleagues (2000). These investigators built network models of the olfactory antennal lobe of the locust. The antennal lobe is a collection of about 800 neurons that relay information from the olfactory receptors to higher brain centers. The antennal lobe has two main dynamical properties. When a stimulus (odor) is presented to the locust, the antennal lobe presents a very fast response. Second, after the odor presentation, the local field potential shows coherent, sustained oscillations. What network architecture would allow such fast and coherent oscillatory response? The authors built networks of Hodgkin–Huxley neurons with different topologies. Regular topology enabled networks to produce coherent oscillations, but the responses were too slow, not in accordance with fast signal processing (Fig. 9.2A). In contrast, networks with random topology could

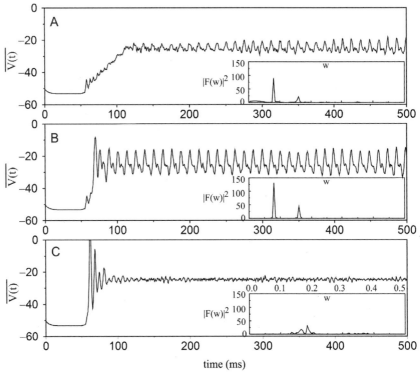

Figure 9.2 **Average activity and power spectrum (inset) in a network of 797 neurons.** (A) Regular network (p = 0). (B) Small-world network (p = 0.032). (C) Random network (p = 1). The input onset occurs at t = 50 ms and is offset at t = 350 ms. Reprinted, with permission, from Lago-Fernandez et al. (2000).

respond very fast, but they were unable to produce coherent activity (Fig. 9.2C). Simple considerations can help to understand the reasons behind these findings. In an ordered network with high local connectivity (high C), it is easy to achieve coherent oscillations, but signals spread very slowly (high L). However, in random networks, signals can spread fast (low L), but, because of the paucity of local connectivity, it is difficult to produce coherent oscillations. However, small world topologies, which possess the best of the ordered and random worlds, can give rise of fast system responses with coherent oscillations (Fig. 9.2B).

As pointed out by Buzsáki and colleagues (2004), functional diversity of interneurons is ideally placed to enhance the computational power of circuits at a low wiring cost. Figure 9.3 illustrates that there is a trade-off between (global) synchronization and wiring economy. In an interneuron-only network of mainly locally connecting basket cells, there is no global synchronization (Fig. 9.3A), although local, transient forms of synchrony can emerge. However, inclusion of even a relatively few long-range interneurons dramatically increases global synchrony, as shown by the emergence of a clear oscillatory rhythm (Fig. 9.3B,C). Figure 9.3D illustrates the relationship between synchrony and wire length. As the fraction of long-range interneurons grows, the synchrony increases, but increasing it above a certain point does not give good return on the investment in wires, since the increase in synchrony becomes more and more modest. Indeed, as illustrated in panel D in Fig. 9.3, there is an optimal portion of long-range interneurons that can give high synchrony with minimal wiring cost.

But are there long-range interneurons in cortical circuits? The question is especially valid in light of the fact that, as mentioned previously, a synonym for interneurons is "local circuit" neurons. For a long time, the generally held belief was that there are only two basic types of interneurons, in terms of their connectivity to principal cells. First, there are those cells, such as the axo-axonic and basket cells, that control principal cell output. Second, there are dendritically projecting interneurons that regulate inputs to principal cells. None of these two general classes of interneurons has particularly long-range connections, especially considering that what we really need are long-range cells that could serve as bona fide shortcuts, connecting distant parts of the network. Unfortunately, a key property of these long-range cells, based on theoretical considerations discussed above in relation to Fig. 9.3, is that they would be expected to be rare, occurring in lower numbers than either the input-controlling, somatically projecting, or the output-regulating, dendritic interneurons. In spite of their predicted rarity, however, several long-range interneuronal subtypes have been found, some somewhat or completely serendipitously, the others as a result of guided searches. Among hippocampal interneurons, the first really long-range interneuronal subtype, discovered in the early 1990s, is a calbindin-containing cell in the stratum oriens with long, horizontally oriented dendrites. The main characteristic of this cell is that it projects from the hippocampus all the way to the medial septum (Toth & Freund, 1992; Toth et al., 1993). Within the medial septum, the axons target mostly GABAergic cells (Toth et al., 1993). Curiously, when the local collaterals of these cells were examined, they also turned out to selectively innervate interneurons (Fig. 9.4) (Gulyás et al, 2003), with the

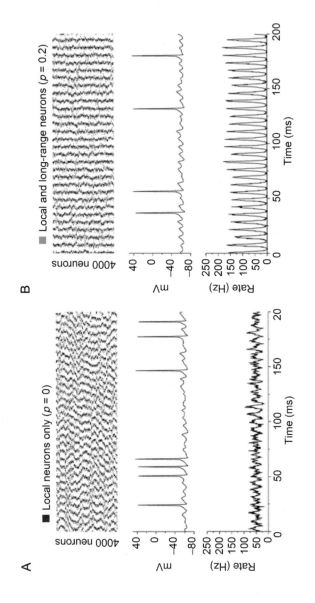

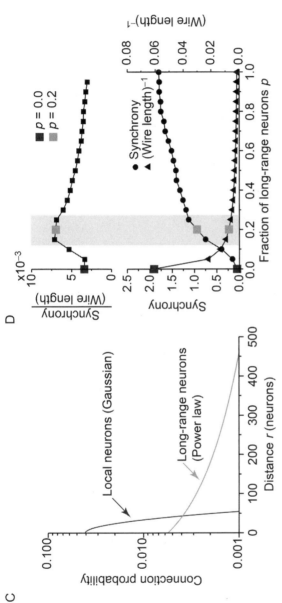

Figure 9.3 **Trade-off between synchronization and wire length economy.** (A) Oscillations in a local network with Gaussian connectivity (characteristic LENGTH=20 neurons). The network is essentially asynchronous. Upper panel, spike raster of 4,000 neurons; middle panel, the voltage trace of a representative neuron; lower panel, the population firing rate. (B) Oscillations in a network with local [Gaussian connectivity as in A] and long-range connections (power-law connectivity). A fraction (20%) of cells contact neurons with a power-law distribution $P(r) \sim (r + k)^{-\alpha}$, where r is the distance between cells, $k = 100$, and $\alpha = 1$. Note clear oscillatory rhythm. (C) Connectivity probability functions: the Gaussian distributed connections are local. With a power distribution, long-range connections become possible. (D) With increasing fraction of long-range neurons p, the network synchrony increases, whereas the inverse of the wire-length of connections decreases (lower panel). Upper panel: An efficiency function is defined as synchrony/length of wire. There is an optimal range of the value p (gray shade) corresponding to high synchrony at a low wire-cost (a small ratio of long-range and short-range connections). Adapted, with permission, from Buzsáki et al. (2004).

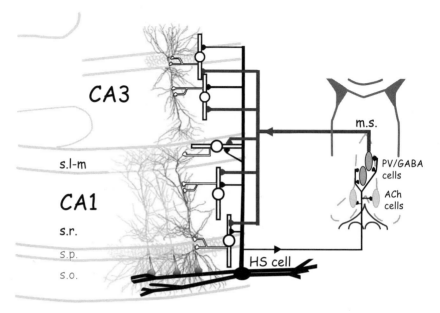

Figure 9.4   **Hippocampo-septal (HS) cells** project both to the medial septum and to remote regions of the hippocampus. Summary diagram illustrates the connections of CA1-HS cells. During highly synchronous principal cell activity, the convergent excitatory drive (shaded gray axon terminals) activates the HS cells. Via their target-selective dual projection, they might synchronize neuronal activity via disinhibition along the septo-hippocampal axis or might silence the medial septum during sharp waves while synchronizing interneurons in the hippocampus. Adapted, with permission, from Gulyás et al. (2003).

axons crossing area boundaries within the hippocampal formation, from CA1 to the CA3 region and to the dentate, as well as from the dorsal (septal) part of the hippocampus to the ventral (temporal part). A third type of hippocampal interneuron that can project to long distances is the previously mentioned "backprojection" interneuron (Sik et al., 1994). This cell's soma was located in CA1, and its vast axons spanned large anatomical areas, including the CA3 and the dentate gyrus. Another type of long-range interneuron resides in the dentate molecular layer projects to the subiculum, connecting the input and output regions of the hippocampal formation (Ceranik et al., 1997; note that CA1 trilaminar cells are also thought to connect to the subiculum, see Fig. 3.1 and related discussion in chapter 3). Thus, without a doubt, there are several types of interneurons that could serve as long-range shortcuts, vastly diminishing the number of nodes (neurons) one has to go through when going from one part to another part of a network.

Real-World Small Worlds: Worming Up to the Hippocampus

But what are the actual L and C values in a real neuronal network? Are these real-world networks truly small world, characterized by low Ls that differ little from the L for an equivalent random network (i.e., a network with the same number of nodes and links as the actual network under scrutiny, but with completely random links between the nodes), and by C values significantly larger than the C calculated for the equivalent random network?

The first L and C calculation for a real, biological neuronal network was performed by Watts and Strogatz (1998). These authors determined the graph structure of the entire nervous system of the worm *Caenorhabditis elegans* (Fig. 9.5). This neuronal network contained about 300 connected neurons (note that only those neurons were considered that could be connected to the "main" graph), where each neuron's identity was known (in fact, each neuron is individually named), and, importantly, the connectivity between the neurons was also precisely established. Watts and Strogatz found that the cells in the nervous system of the worm were connected in a manner that corresponded to the small world network graphs, characterized by a low L and a high C (Fig. 9.5). Furthermore, the low L was similar to the L for an equivalent random graph, whereas the C determined for the worm nervous system was considerably higher than the C for the random network. The low L in the worm's nervous system indicated that the network was globally well-connected, as it took less than three steps to reach any neuron from any neuron on average. In contrast, the high C indicated that the network was also well-connected locally (i.e., the neurons formed local clusters whose members were especially heavily interlinked).

But what do we know about the L and C of real mammalian networks? Here, the task is much harder. First, there are many more neurons, as well as many distinct neuronal types, and the identity and connectivity of the individual neurons in mammalian networks are obviously not known with the same precision as in the worm, making the task of establishing L and C much harder. However, a good deal

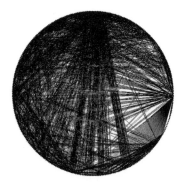

	L_{actual}	L_{random}	C_{actual}	C_{random}
C elegans	2.65	2.25	0.28	0.05

Figure 9.5 **Small-world networks and the graph structure of the nervous system of C. ele-gans.** Cells were arranged in a circle, and the synaptic connections were indicated by links (data generously supplied by Dr Watts, from the same database as in Watts and Strogatz, 1998). At the bottom of the graph, the L and C values for the nervous system of the worm is shown, as well as the L and C values for the equivalent random graphs (containing the same number of nodes and links). Reprinted, with permission, from Földy et al. (2005).

of data has been gathered over the years about the elements and connectivity rules for many mammalian microcircuits in various brain regions. The rodent dentate gyrus, in particular, has been especially well studied, due to its role in limbic information processing as well as in a whole variety of neurological disorders, such as ischemia, epilepsy and head trauma.

The rodent dentate gyrus contains two excitatory and at least six distinct types of interneurons (see Table 7.1; note that the number of interneuronal species in the dentate is almost certainly higher and will increase with future research, but these are the ones that we currently know about, in terms of solid anatomical and physiological data). The excitatory cells are the granule cells and the mossy cells, whereas the interneurons consist of the basket, axo-axonic, HIPP, MOPP, HICAP, and IS cells (see Table 7.1 for details) (Santhakumar & Soltesz, 2004; Földy et al., 2005). It is interesting to consider their numbers and their "links" (a single link here signifies the presence of a synaptic connection, irrespective of its strength or whether the connection between the two cell types has a single or multiple contacts; note also that the links are directed connections, just like synaptic contacts). The rat dentate gyrus contains about a million cells, with the majority of them (94%) being granule cells. These million neurons are connected by over a billion links, with the majority of these links being excitatory, glutamatergic. The "relational graph" (i.e., a graph indicating the relationship between the different types of nodes, where a link just indicates that a connection is known to exist, irrespective of its frequency of occurrence) shows that the different cell types are densely interconnected (note that only <1% of the connections are actually between neurons of the same type) (Dyhrfjeld-Johnsen et al., 2004). Interestingly, there is a large difference in the degrees of interconnectedness between the different neuronal species. For example, mossy cells (a type of glutamatergic non-principal cell in the hilus) form the highest number of outputs (more than 30,000 per a single mossy cell), but the numerically most frequent cells, the granule cells, give the fewest contacts (only about 200 "nodes" are linked from a single granule cell) (Dyhrfjeld-Johnsen et al., 2004). A crucial difference between estimating the L and C for the worm nervous system and the mammalian dentate is that, in the latter case, the topographic axon distributions must also be taken into account. In simple terms, the rat dentate gyrus is an approximately 6mm long, elongated structure, and neurons have a restricted spatial range for their axon arbors that is generally smaller than the length of the dentate gyrus. Consequently, a granule cell in position x along the septo-temporal axis of the hippocampus contacts nearby mossy cells with a different probability than mossy cells that are located some distance away, and similar location-dependency applies to all cell types. Luckily, a lot is known about the spatial distributions of axons of the various cell types, from in vivo single cell filling experiments that allowed the reconstruction of the whole axonal arbors of various cells, and it has been shown that the axonal arbors could be well fitted with either a single Gaussian, or two partially overlapping Gaussians (Dyhrfjeld-Johnsen et al., 2004). A key feature of the topographic connections is that granule cell axons are the spatially most restricted. The axonal tree of a single granule cell spans about 600 µm in the septo-temporal direction (note that the definition of a hippocampal lamella is precisely the span of a single mossy fiber, i.e., the axon of a single granule cell). In contrast, the axonal arbor of a single mossy cell spans almost the entire dentate gyrus. The axonal spans of interneurons (note that we are concerned here exclusively with the intradentate connections, not with long-distance connections between different hippocampal and other brain areas) tend to be somewhere in between the spatially most restricted granule cell axons and the spatially most extensive mossy cell axons. It is a curious fact, which will play prominently later on in our discussions, that the cells with the longest links (mossy cells, followed by the HIPP and HICAP interneurons) are also the ones that are selectively lost in epilepsy. As far as the healthy, control graph structure is concerned, the conclusion from these data is that we have cells that are essentially local in terms of their connectivity, and cells that may serve as long-distance links within the dentate gyrus.

Armed with these cell type-specific connectivity and axonal topography data, it became possible, for the first time, to determine the L and C values for a real-life mammalian neuronal network, by building a computer representation of the neuronal graph (Dyhrfjeld-Johnsen et al., 2004). Initially, glutamatergic and GABAergic links were considered the same way (note that both types of contacts can serve as mechanisms of synchronization in the network; of course, the two types of links can also be separated later). The first surprise was that the L for the entire dentate gyrus, with its more than a million nodes and billion links, still had an extremely low average path length. In fact, the L (2.6) for the dentate gyrus turned out to be virtually identical to the L calculated by Watts and Strogatz (1998) for the worm nervous system. The second important observation was that the L for the dentate network was only slightly higher than the L calculated for the equivalent random graph (2.25), indicating the small-world nature of the dentate circuit. In support of the latter conclusion, the C of the dentate was almost 25 times higher than the C calculated for the equivalent random network (Dyhrfjeld-Johnsen et al., 2004). These data, for the first time, established that mammalian neuronal circuits are indeed bona fide small-world networks.

Of course, it should be kept in mind that, although the dentate gyrus may be the whole world to its dedicated enthusiasts, it still represents only a part of the hippocampal formation, and an even smaller part of the whole mammalian central nervous system. Although it will take additional studies to establish the L and C values for larger mammalian networks, we can already make educated guesses. For example, it is likely that the low L values calculated in the Dyrhfjeld-Johnsen et al. (2004) study for the dentate gyrus will not increase much when larger parts of the rodent central nervous system are considered, precisely because of those extremely long-distant connections that we discussed in the previous section. For example, we know that long-range interneurons in the dentate gyrus can reach as far as the subiculum (Ceranik et al., 1997) or the septum (Gulyás et al., 2003). Thus, it would take only one or two additional steps to reach other brain areas from the dentate gyrus. Once we reach those distant areas using the super-long connections, local links will likely allow us to reach any other neuron from a few steps, assuming that the L and C values calculated for the dentate gyrus are representative of other brain areas as well. It should also be noted that several studies calculated the L values between brain areas (Stephan et al., 2000; Sporns & Zwi, 2004; Striedter, 2005) (note that in these latter studies, entire cortical areas were considered nodes, and axonal projections between them were considered direct links). The L determined in this "macro" way turned out to be low, supporting the prediction that the L and C values determined for the entire mammalian brain will be commensurate with a solidly small world architectural design.

Attack Tolerance of Small-World Networks: Hippocampal Sclerosis as a Natural Experiment

The low L in the worm's nervous system and in the mammalian dentate gyrus indicated that both networks were globally well-connected, as it took less than three steps to reach any neuron from any neuron on average. In contrast, the high C values suggested that the circuits were also well-connected locally (i.e., the neurons formed local clusters whose members were heavily interlinked). As discussed above, small-world network topology allows both fast computations in local microcircuits and the efficient relay of signals to distant parts of the network, with the potential for global synchronization of activity patterns. Thus, in essence, a high C can underlie a special propensity for local synchrony and fast local computations, whereas a low L allows activity to easily spread throughout the network, leading to global synchrony (Lago-Fernandez et al. 2000; Barahona & Pecora 2002; Li & Chen 2003; Masuda & Aihara 2004). Recent modeling studies also indicated that changes in L and C can strongly modulate the action potential discharge patterns (e.g., tonic firing versus bursting) in model CA1 and CA3 networks (Netoff et al., 2004).

Given the current knowledge about the functional relevance of small-world structure in neuronal networks, can we make any predictions as to what happens to neuronal circuits in the face of attacks that delete nodes and links from the graph? A well-known phenomenon is hippocampal end-folium (an early name for the dentate gyrus) sclerosis, where, during epileptogenesis, recurrent seizures in the limbic system result in the death of more and more hilar cells, which, in turn, is thought to trigger more and more sprouting of mossy fibers (the axons of granule cells). Maximal sclerosis takes place when all hilar cells are lost (these include the mossy, HIPP, HICAP and IS cells; see Table 7.1 and Fig. 7.1) and mossy fiber sprouting reaches its peak, which is thought to be about 300 extra mossy fiber contacts per granule cell (Buckmaster & Dudek, 1999; Buckmaster et al., 2002; see also Santhakumar et al., 2005). Simple calculations show that the loss of all hilar cells and maximal sprouting leads to a rather small decrease in the total number of neurons (<5%), but there is a massive loss of links from the network (74% of the 1.2 billion links are lost) (Dyhfjeld-Johnsen et al., 2004). Given this dramatic reduction in intrinsic connections, one may expect the collapse of the small-world network topology in the dentate gyrus. In order to gain a precise view of what happens as sclerosis progresses, L and C were calculated for various degrees of sclerosis. These calculations showed that sclerosis (i.e., the loss of hilar cells and mossy fiber sprouting) did not cause a significant increase in L until almost all hilar cells were lost. This may seem surprising at first, however, this observation perfectly matches what Watts and Strogatz (1998) found, namely, that even a few long-distance connections are sufficient to keep L low. Furthermore, the relative L (L for the dentate network divided by the L for the equivalent random graph; the relative L should be close to unity for a small-world network) actually decreased, progressively approaching unity during most of the sclerosis. In fact, the relative L increased only right before the onset of full sclerosis. Thus, these data indicated that there was a great deal of stability in terms of the preservation of the basic small-world architecture of the dentate network, and that even massive loss of links did not result in the collapse of the small-world networks, as long as at least a few hilar cells are left. Importantly, the changes in C values with sclerosis were in agreement with these conclusions. The changes in relative C indicated that the progression of sclerosis resulted in an enhancement of the small-world features of the network (high C, compared to the equivalent random network), and that it was only with the onset of severe sclerosis (90% hilar cell loss and mossy fiber sprouting) that the relative C values dipped below the control C value obtained for the healthy network (Dyhrfjeld-Johnsen et al., 2004). Further analysis revealed that the sprouting of mossy fibers onto granule cells is the major factor underlying the changes in network topology during the earlier phases of sclerosis, as mossy fiber sprouting keeps the path length low and leads to the increases in C. Due to the large number of hilar cell connections to granule cells, the effects of mild to moderate hilar cell loss on L and C are essentially counteracted by local mossy fiber sprouting. Once the sclerosis exceeds 90%, the loss of hilar cells becomes the defining factor, but, as long as at least a fraction of the highly connected, long-distance hilar cells survive, they can sustain the small-world structure of the dentate gyrus. Note that various interneuronal species, with their characteristic axonal trees, substantially contribute to the L and C values in the healthy networks, as well as to the shapes of the plots of L and C changes with the progression of sclerosis (e.g., the increase in C during the initial phases of sclerosis, due to the setting up of new connections between granule cell pairs that were connected to the same non-granule cell, is larger and more prolonged in a network with interneurons present than in the isolated excitatory network; Dyhrfjeld-Johsen et al., 2004). In fact, it is quite possible that the role of interneurons in shaping changes in L and C may be recognized to be even larger in the future, as interneuronal axons may also undergo sprouting in certain pathological conditions. More quantitative data on GABAergic sprouting will be needed to establish which interneuronal species (e.g., types with primarily local, mid- or long-range axonal arbors) undergo sprouting following repeated seizures and injury.

But what is the functional relevance of the changes in the small-world network architecture during end-folium sclerosis? Based on previous studies, small-world topology should generally enhance long-distance signal propagation and synchrony. Thus, the straightforward prediction is that, in the absence of other changes (e.g., in synaptic strengths), epileptiform activity should initially increase, but, with the loss of the last long-range links form the hilus, the degree of seizure-like activity should show a decrease. This is a somewhat counterintuitive proposition, as more advanced hippocampal sclerosis is generally taken to signify the presence of more seizures.

This paradoxical prediction was tested in a large-scale, anatomically and biophysically realistic network model that contained 50,000 granule cells, 1,500 mossy cells, 500 basket cells, and 600 HIPP cells (for other interneurons, there was not enough detailed information available to build detailed, multicompartmental single-cell models; note that each model cell closely reproduced the experimentally determined firing rates and firing patterns, and was connected with realistic excitatory or inhibitory synaptic couplings; for details, see Santhakumar et al., 2005). Importantly, the graph of the model network reproduced the L and C changes that take place in the biological, real network with sclerosis. The amount of firing in the network was minimal in the healthy network with zero sclerosis, and the degree of excitability, as well as the speed of the propagation of the activity, increased progressively with the advancement of sclerosis. However, beyond a certain point with severe sclerosis, the degree of hyperactivity started to dip, exactly as predicted based on the changes in small-world network structure. Thus, in spite of the presence of maximal mossy fiber sprouting with 100% sclerosis, maximal sclerosis did not represent a maximally permissive circuit structure for epilepsy. Local synchrony could still develop with severe sclerosis, but the local activity had to propagate at a slower, piecemeal fashion, from lamella to lamella, in the absence of long-range connections.

Scale-Free Networks: Interneurons as Hubs

Many systems can be depicted as networks with complex topologies. The connection topology, initially assumed to be either ordered (regular) or random by Erdös and Rényi (1960), was shown by Watts and Strogatz (1998) to include a new class of network topologies that lie in between the two extremes, as discussed above. As also mentioned above, several biological, technological, and social networks, including the power grid of the western United States, the sociological networks of collaborating mathematicians, the casting of actors in movies, and neuronal networks, can all be shown to be of the small-world type (Watts & Strogatz, 1998). Formally, a small-world graph can be defined as a sparse graph that is much more highly clustered than an equally sparse random graph (Wuchty, 2001). Although these ideas from Watts and Strogatz proved to be extremely fertile, and resulted in a number of major insights in a wide variety of scientific disciplines (Buchanan, 2002), they did not fully capture all the defining features of complex networks.

It was in 1999 that the physicists Albert-László Barabási and Réka Albert published a paper that suddenly revealed a whole new class of networks, the so-called scale-free networks. They studied growing networks, unlike the essentially stationary networks considered by Watts and Strogatz (1998). There were only two rules necessary to generate these networks. First, the networks were allowed to expand continuously, with the addition of new nodes (or "vertices"). Second, the newly added nodes attached preferentially to nodes that were already well-connected. Thus, this was essentially a "rich-gets-richer" scheme. An important consequence of this generic growth mechanism was that it invariably resulted in a connectivity distribution that decayed according to a power-law, characterized by a few extremely well-connected "hubs." Note that the power-law distribution implies that the number of links per node, k, obeys a power law, that is, $P(k) \sim k^{\alpha}$ (in other words, the number of nodes with exactly k links follows this power law for any value of k), where the degree exponent a is usually around 2 to 3. This is a heavily skewed distribution, with a few nodes possessing an exceptionally high number of links. Because this feature was independent of network size, this class of inhomogeneous networks was named "scale-free" networks (Fig. 9.6). In a sense, the presence of a few major connectors, which possessed an unusually large number of links, gave the networks an aristocratic character (Buchanan, 2002), as opposed to the more egalitarian node-link distribution of the networks considered by Watts and Strogatz (1998). Subsequently, numerous real-life networks were shown to be scale-free networks. For example, the topology of the Web can be constructed by considering the HTML documents as the nodes and the connections between them as the links pointing from one page to another (Albert et al., 1999; Barabási & Albert, 1999; Barabási et al al., 2000). The resulting topology clearly demonstrated scale-free properties, with certain popular Web pages (such as Yahoo! or cnn.com) serving as major hubs, whereas others (such as, sadly, the Web pages of even the most illustrious interneuronal researchers) possessing only a few links. Several biological networks were also shown to display scale-free characteristics, for example, the metabolic networks of various organisms, with substrates as nodes and the directed links symbolizing the biochemical reactions (Fell & Wagner, 2000; Jeong et al., 2000). The hubs in this

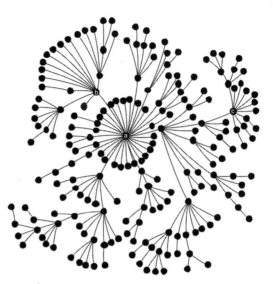

Figure 9.6 **Schematic illustration of a scale-free graph,** grown by attaching new nodes at random to previously existing nodes. The probability of attachment is proportional to the degree of the target node; thus richly connected nodes tend to get richer, leading to the formation of hubs and a skewed degree distribution with a heavy tail. Letters indicate the three nodes with the most links (a, k = 33 links; b, k = 12; c, k = 11). Here, n = 200 nodes, m = 199 links. Adapted, with permission, from Strogatz (2001).

latter case were certain molecules involved in an extremely large number of biochemical reactions, such as coenzyme A, pyruvate, and glutamate. Interestingly, the average path length ("diameter") of the biochemical networks was not only low, but it also remained largely identical regardless of the number of substrates found in the studied organisms, chiefly because one can easily reach any node from any node in different parts of the network by going through the richly connected hubs. Thus, because of the hubs, the scale-free networks are also small-world networks (but not all small-world networks are scale-free). It is useful to bring in a human example again, in order to gain an intuitive sense of what the scale-free networks are about. When Mark Newman (2001) studied the statistics of Medline to reveal rules underlying the patterns of collaborations among scientists, he found that "the probability of a particular scientist acquiring new collaborators increases with the number of his or her past collaborators" (see also Buchanan, 2002). Again, the rich gets richer, in this case, because the perceived benefit of collaborating with someone apparently increases if that person already has many published collaborative studies. The key point is that preferential attachment of new nodes to already well-connected nodes leads to a particular network structure, the scale-free architecture, characterized by a vast number of sparsely connected nodes and a few extremely richly connected ones.

But do these scale-free ideas also apply to neuronal networks? In principle, one could imagine a situation where newly added neurons during development preferentially attach to neurons that are already well-connected, which should result in a scale-free network. However, the available hard data do not entirely support this proposition. For example, the neuronal network of the worm is fairly egalitarian, it has no true hubs, as each neuron is linked to about 14 others. Similarly, no scale-free, power law–abiding architecture was found in the neuronal network of the mammalian dentate gyrus (Dyhrfjeld-Johnsen et al., 2004). In the latter case, frequency distribution of the number of links (incoming or outgoing or both) revealed the relatively poorly connected granule cells forming one massively dominant peak, followed by a few minor peaks on the right representing the better-connected other cell types. However, there was no evidence of the existence of true "connectors" or "hubs" that would follow a strict power-law distribution (note that these data focused on the intrinsic connections of the dentate gyrus only). Although future research may reveal neurons which serve as hubs, the fact is that, at least in the case of the two microcircuits (where neurons are the nodes and synaptic connections are the links, as opposed to entire brain areas being considered as nodes) from which hard data have been obtained (Watts & Strogatz, 1998; Dyhrfjeld-Johnsen et al., 2004), there is no evidence of scale-free networks.

An interesting suggestion put forward by Mark Buchanan (2002) is that certain limitations may explain why in some systems scale-free architecture cannot develop. Namely, it is suggested that perhaps it becomes too expensive to add still more links to a single node to individual neurons, limiting the maximal number of synaptic links. Although this is certainly an attractive idea, and it may even apply to the worm as well as the dentate gyrus, it should be pointed out that most neurons, typically, would seem to be able to receive more synapses on their surfaces and may be able to make more synapses (note that the surfaces of mammalian neurons are not completely covered by synapses, in fact, it is a common observation in the electron microscope that a large part of the neuronal surface is free from synaptic inputs; of course, there could be other, e.g., energetic, limitations for increasing synaptic coverage).

However, all this does not mean that the scale-free ideas are not applicable in some form to neuronal networks. In fact, these ideas are extremely powerful in providing us with new insights, even if the actual biological neuronal networks do not perfectly conform to the power-law distribution. For example, it is clear that, as mentioned above, certain neuronal species in the dentate gyrus are more connected than others, and that, curiously, it is the more vulnerable cell types that form the most far-reaching axonal arbors and possess high numbers of connections, such as the mossy cells and HIPP cells. Furthermore, the ideas of Barabási and Albert focus our attention on the long-range interneurons that connect different brain areas. Barabási and colleagues in a further study showed that scale-free networks are very resistant to random attack, where nodes are removed by chance, but these same networks are, in fact, extremely vulnerable to directed attacks that specifically target the connectors, the most richly connected hubs (Albert et al., 2000). These studies revealed the fundamental importance of network topology in determining the robustness of the network in response to random deletions and targeted attacks. Communication networks display frequent malfunctions of various components, but local failures rarely result in a total collapse of the information-carrying capacity of the global network (Albert et al., 2000). Although redundancy in wiring plays a role in such error-tolerance phenomena, another important factor is the inhomogeneous network topology; that is, the small-world and scale-free topologies (Buzsáki et al., 2004). In the case of many real networks, such as the World Wide Web, the Internet, social networks, and metabolic networks, such tolerance to random removal of nodes comes at the high price of being very sensitive to targeted attacks that specifically delete the most heavily interconnected nodes (Albert et al., 2000). A particularly illuminating example of the importance of such topological approaches came from the demonstration that, in a protein–protein interaction network from the yeast, the likelihood that the removal of a protein will prove lethal strongly correlates with the number of interactions the protein has, or, in other words, the most highly connected proteins are the most important for the cell's survival (Jeong et al., 2001).

These insights are, of course, highly relevant for the understanding the role of interneuronal loss in neurological diseases. If the long-distance, well-connected interneuronal species are specifically vulnerable to certain insults, they may drastically reduce the internal connectivity of the neuronal networks, even if the networks in which these interneurons reside do not perfectly conform to scale-free networks. In fact, we have already mentioned above that the loss of hilar cells (mossy cells and HIPP cells) dramatically reduces the number of intrinsic connections within the dentate gyrus. If we considered not only the dentate gyrus, but several other related brain areas as well, these long-distant interneuronal species are becoming especially intriguing in terms of their contribution to the sensitivity of the network to targeted attacks. For example, it is possible that after traumatic brain injury (e.g., after a severe concussion), neurons with long connections may be especially subjected to shear forces and traveling pressure wave-transients, which could result in their preferential injury. Whether this is the case is not yet known, but it is clear that the revolutionary ideas of Barabási and Albert allowed us to be able to ask these questions, and determine in future experiments whether, for example, the hippocampo-septal hilar interneurons are preferentially lost after trauma, seizures, or ischemia. As an added benefit, these studies will also help us to evaluate whether certain rare interneuronal species serve as hubs in the neuronal networks of the neocortex and hippocampus.

Interneuronal Heterogeneity in Small-World Networks

In summary, it is clear that there is a close, albeit not fully understood relationship between interneuronal heterogeneity and small-world architecture. Regarding the species diversity aspect of interneuronal heterogeneity, it seems plausible that the functional diversity of interneurons augments computational power at a low wiring cost (Buzsáki et a., 2004). Some interneuronal species are more interconnected than others to similar or different cell types. For example, axo-axonic cells do not or rarely innervate each other or other types of interneurons, whereas basket cells make contacts on proximal basket cells and other interneuronal species (Sik et al., 1995; Katsumaru et al., 1988; Tamas et al., 2000). Several dendritically projecting interneuronal species are known to be interconnected within the same population, and also contact axo-axonic and basket cells (Sik et al., 1997; Buzsáki et al., 2004). Although it seems that interneuronal networks do not contain a truly "superhub" species that would be represented by only a few individuals carrying a disproportional part of the total connections, the differential degree of connectivity for the various interneuronal species, together with the highly specific wiring, can support numerous flexible functions (Watts & Strogatz, 1998; Barabási, 2002; Changizi, 2003; Buzsáki et al., 2004). As suggested by Buzsáki and colleagues (2004), interactions between different interneuronal species may support global oscillations at different frequencies (Csicsvary et al., 1999; Pike et al., 2000; Whittington et al., 2000; Whittington & Traub, 2003) and may also be conducive to synaptic plasticity (Miles et al., 1996; Buzsáki et al., 1996; Maccaferri et al., 1998; Traub et al., 1998). As mentioned above, it is a straightforward prediction from theoretical considerations and modeling (Fig 9.3) that interneurons with only local connectivity should be the most numerous, whereas those interneuronal species that typically have widespread connections should be the least numerous (Buzsáki et al., 2004). Figure 9.7 shows this hypothesis explicitly. Perisomatic interneurons should be the most numerous, followed by the specific (single) and less-specific (multiple) dendrite-innervating subtypes. Therefore, the vast majority of interneuronal wiring should be local, and cells with a more global impact should be rarer. The figure also illustrates a predicted scaling relationship between interneurons depending on the physical size of the neuronal network. According to this interesting prediction, the slope of the functions in the figure (the ratio of interneurons with local and distant connectivity) should be higher for larger brain areas (e.g., neocortex versus hippocampus). Although these predictions need to be tested in future studies, the fact that we can now put forward and consider such explicit, quantitative relationships indicate that the field of interneuronal microcircuit research is rapidly gaining an unprecedented level of maturity, where ideas from vastly different disciplines can be integrated to provide new insights into the functional architecture of microcircuits.

The relationship of the other aspect of interneuronal heterogeneity, intraspecies variance, with the ideas of small-world topology of neuronal networks is also not entire understood. As discussed above, a plot of the number of incoming or outgoing links for the intrinsic connections between the various glutamatergic and GABAergic cells in the dentate gyrus revealed one dominant peak, followed by several sparsely spaced, much smaller peaks on the right

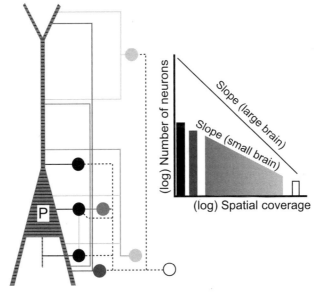

Figure 9.7   **A hypothetical connection scheme of cortical interneurons.** Connections and cell-body locations are based on information gathered in the hippocampus (P, principal neuron). The graph shows a hypothesized relationship between spatial coverage and the number of neurons in a given class. Perisomatic (black) interneurons with small spatial coverage are most numerous, whereas long-range interneurons (open) that interconnect different regions are few. Many other classes (shades of gray) might occupy an intermediate coverage. The slope of this hypothesized relationship should vary with network size. With increasing brain size, the number of interneurons with local connections increases more rapidly than neurons with more extensive spatial coverage. The power law shown here is for illustration purposes only, to indicate that a mathematically defined relationship might exist between spatial coverage and number of neurons in particular interneuron classes. Adapted, with permission, from Buzsáki et al. (2004).

of the granule cell peak, without revealing a bona fide power-law distribution (Dyhrfjeld-Johnsen et al., 2004). The width of each peak in this plot reveals the degree of cell-to-cell variability in the number of incoming or outgoing links. Unfortunately, this is the kind of information that proves to be the scarcest in the literature, as most publications are based on relatively few reconstructed cells (understandably, given the amount of work involved), and, therefore, the cell-to-cell variability in the connectivity patterns of the various cellular species is difficult to ascertain. However, because the approximate mean values for the average number of links have been estimated (Dyhrfjeld-Johnsen et al., 2004), one can artificially vary the spread to the (presumed) Gaussian around each peak.

Interestingly, even if the spread is extremely large, so that the individual Gaussians overlap, the resulting distribution still fails to provide a true power-law distribution. As mentioned before, however, it should be kept in mind that these results are only for the intrinsic connections of one mammalian brain region, the dentate gyrus. It is still possible that, when larger brain regions will be considered, with the long-range interneurons also taken into account, the resulting graph topology may conform not only to the small world structure (Watts & Strogatz, 1998; Dyhrfjeld-Johnsen et al., 2004), but it may also reveal a hitherto unimagined, perhaps completely novel neuronal network architecture.

10

Closing Thoughts: The Structure of Cortical Microcircuit Theory

----

Truth emerges more readily from error than from confusion.
                                        T. S. Kuhn (1996)

Resolution of the Diversity Debate

The astonishing heterogeneity of interneurons has kindled a great deal of research that led to a variety of conclusions regarding the origins and functions of interneuronal heterogeneity. On the one hand, there have been many examples of an almost crystal-like order in the organization of interneurons. Reports of data that supported the exquisite order in interneuronal heterogeneity were intellectually reassuring (and frequently esthetically pleasing), as they pointed to the fulfillment of Cajal's paradigm as the clear end-point toward which research should progress. On the other hand, there has also been a steady stream of studies that reported only weak or nonexistent correlations and imperfect mapping between certain experimentally determined parameters and interneuronal classes, emphasizing (and perhaps overemphasizing) the presence of variability in interneuronal populations. Although some of the latter class of results could always be critized by arguments that alleged some technical reasons for the less than crystalline outcome, the persistently recurring nature of these studies were nevertheless worrisome, as they signaled difficulties ahead for further progress based on the narrowly interpreted Cajal paradigm. It is an interesting point for future neuroscience historians to explore that high-profile reports of even the most implausible degrees of perfection in interneuronal microcircuits seemed to be often immune from criticisms evoking experimental errors for the reported outcome, perhaps because positive findings of an immaculate order have an inherent esthetic appeal over negative findings.

In this book, a resolution of this "diversity debate" was outlined that ventured beyond the passive acceptance of the unavoidable existence of some mystical order–disorder dichotomy in complex biological systems. As emphasized throughout the book, it is crucial to clearly differentiate heterogeneity, variability, and diversity, as a great deal of the disagreements in the literature arose from the mixing of arguments related to cell-to-cell variability within defined interneuronal subtypes with data on interneuronal species diversity. In addition, it was argued that cell-to-cell variability not only naturally existed within populations of interneurons belonging to the same subtype, but that this cell-to-cell variability had several functional consequences, including regulation of neuronal excitability, oscillatory activity, and network synchrony. We also suggested that, given the significant functional effects of altered variability from both modeling and experimental studies, the extent of cell-to-cell variability is likely to be regulated by a variety of developmental factors, subcortical neuromodulators, and perhaps also by the external environment. Finally, it was also pointed out that cell-to-cell variability may be a consequence of the homeostatic processes, with each neuron finding a particular "solution" to its given function in the circuit. Quantitative techniques to compare variability (e.g., with the Conover test) and assess interneuronal diversity (with the Shanon–Wiener diversity index) were also discussed, to enable future comparisons of data on interneuronal heterogeneity. Taken together, these results hopefully will not only generate more cutting-edge research in the field, but will also lead to more clarity in future discussions regarding interneuronal heterogeneity, variability, and diversity.

Building a Complex Machine from Variable Parts

The bulk of the available structural and functional data on interneurons clearly shows that distinct interneuronal species exist in cortical neuronal circuits, each with its specific, characteristic properties and functional roles. However, the existence of distinct interneuronal species does not mean that real-life, biological neuronal networks are constructed from a finite set of homogeneous pieces, like a mechanical machine from screws, cogwheels, and nuts and bolts. The variability of the parts, we argued, constituted a key characteristic of neuronal systems, as the degree of variance strongly modulates how the networks behave under a variety of circumstances.

With the significant recent progress in our knowledge about interneuronal anatomy and physiology on the one hand, and computational neuroscience on the other, it is increasingly feasible to build biologically realistic, large-scale network models (e.g., Dyhrfjeld-Johnsen et al., 2004; Traub et al., 2004; Hill & Tononi, 2005; Santhakumar et al., 2005). During the construction of these computational network models, as a first step, single-cell models for each of the neuronal cell types present in the particular brain area are built, usually based on averaged, mean data from a number of laboratories. However, the cell-to-cell variability for the various parameters is not taken into account explicitly, for at least two reasons. First, in many cases, the cell-to-cell variability is usually not reported in the literature. Second, implementation of the cell-to-cell variability for each of the numerous parameters is computationally complex. As a compromise, in many models, a certain amount of variability is introduced artificially, most often by a slight dispersion of a tonic inward current among the cells. To what extent this method actually approximates the real effects of cell-to-cell variability among interneurons is not well understood, but it is clear that it cannot represent the full array of functional consequences of variability. The reason for this is simple. Namely, the level of cell-to-cell variability is likely to be different for the various parameters (e.g., calcium currents, sodium currents, etc.), and the degree of dispersion for any one parameter is also likely to be dynamically changing, perhaps due to ascending neuromodulatory influences. Hopefully, with the recognition of the importance of the naturally occurring variability within distinct interneuronal populations, more data will become reported in this regard, which will enable the construction of large-scale computational network models that incorporate cell-to-cell variability data for interneuronal subgroups in the future. Parallel to these efforts aimed at understanding the normal degree of variability among interneuronal populations, attention should be paid to determining whether cell-to-cell variability undergoes short- and long-term alterations in various neurological disease models, in addition to simple decreases in interneuronal diversity through cell loss in trauma and epilepsy.

Phenogenetic Perspective for Interneuronal Research and the Role of Chance

In several places in this book, analogies with evolution and ecosystem theory were employed to provide us with tools and approaches toward understanding interneuronal microcircuits. For example, we took advantage of certain analogies between interneuronal subtypes and animal and plant species, applied the diversity index from ecosystem analysis to quantitatively measure species diversity, envisioned Linnean classification systems for interneurons, and raised the specter of ontogenetic cladistics for interneurons. In addition, we have discussed the evolutionary angles of interneuronal heterogeneity, as they relate to inheritable traits and behavior, explored the developmental origins of interneuronal species and intra-subtype variability, and argued that certain variations among individual cells belonging to any given interneuronal species objectively exist and are not inconsequential, a statement that bears an unmistakeable resemblance to evolutionary theory. An obvious question is whether there is a deeper link between evolutionary theory and interneuronal heterogeneity, and between ecosystem and cortical microcircuit organization, beyond the apparent usefulness of analogies and the intellectual delight one may take in catapulting back and forth across the alluring, sweeping vistas of the uninhabited canyonlands separating these seemingly distant fields of biology?

In fact, the question has a broad relevance to arguably the greatest puzzle in contemporary biology, which is how the astonishing diversity of biological traits is produced by a linear sequence of nucleotides (Weiss, 2005). Although Charles Darwin and Alfred Wallace produced a powerful explanation of how life works through changes in the frequency of variations, even the later forms of evolutionary theory incorporating population genetics could not explain how genes produce the complex traits that characterize organisms. An emergening, more complete evolutionary synthesis, called evolution of development or "EvoDevo," aims to reveal the phenogenetic logic or relational principles of life, explaining how a few basic characteristics of genomes can produce complex phenotypes through some fundamental developmental processes. As explained eloquently in a particularly elegant article on the subject by Kenneth Weiss (2005),

> Phenogenetic logic can be encapsulated by the general principle of duplication with variation, driven by change in gene expression, component sequestration, functional divergence and chance. The symmetry between phenogenetic logic and Darwin's principles is not accidental (Table 10.1). If evolution is the history of species, phenogenetics is history within organisms. Species evolution and embryological development are both nested phenomena of differentiation between units — organisms in species evolution, and cells or gene products in development.

The arguments summarized in Table 10.1 suggest, therefore, that there is justification for keeping a close eye on the symmetries between evolution and phenogenetics to help explain both the order and variability in interneuronal microcircuits. A full understanding of the emergence of interneuronal species through development will require the determination of "sources of variation" (differential gene expression) (note that the expression "sources of variation" in Table 10.1 would be closer to "sources of diversity" according to the definitions of terms used in this book), and the "means of divergence" (functional specialization through programmed responses to signaling and other internal conditions). To look at the other side of Janus' face, however, we will also need to take into account the role of chance in the emergence of interneuronal heterogeneity. It is well-known that chance is critical in the generation of evolutionary change, but chance also has widespread, albeit less understood roles in development as well. The key role of chance is well-appreciated in the somatic recombination in mammalian antibody genes, but chance, as Table 10.1 indicates, may also play a variety of other roles, through the molecular stochasticity of regulatory components, somatic mutations, and epigenetic modifications of promoter regions. In several places throughout this book, we have highlighted these potentially important sources of interneuronal intraspecies variability, but it is clear that much more needs to be done to integrate the perspectives and findings of phenogenetics and interneuronal order and heterogeneity.

It is interesting to note here that some of the central ideas discussed in this book also share a certain amount common ground

Table 10.1 Comparative logic and symmetries between evolution and phenogenetics.

Characteristic	Evolution	Phenogenetics
Overall principle	Descent with modification	Duplication with variation
Explains	Life through the history of organisms	Life through form and function, a somatic history within organisms
Source of variation	Gametic mutation	Differential gene expression
Means of sequestration	Mating barriers and speciation through mechanisms of genomic and ecological isolation	Partial sequestration with information transfer through signaling using arbitrary codes
Means of divergence	Adaptation by competitive response to external conditions	Functional specialization through programmed response to signaling and other internal conditions
Role of chance	Genetic drift	Molecular stochasticity in timing and concentration of components, somatic mutation, and epigenetic modification (e.g., methylation).

Reprinted, with permission, from Weiss (2005)

with, and may have implications for, a global theory of brain function called neuronal Darwinism. This theory, alternatively known as the theory of neuronal group selection (Edelman, 1993), emphasized the role of population thinking and variations between cells. One of the three tenets of this theory is developmental selection, where epigenetic variations in the precise details of the connections between developing neurons create repertoires of local circuits in each brain area. Developmental selection, together with the other two tenets of the theory, experiential selection and reentry, form a selectional system that is analogous to other selectional systems including evolution and the immune system. All of these selectional systems function according to three main principles (Edelman, 1993, 2004). First, there has to be a means for generating variations in a population of elements (individual animals, cells, or molecules). The second principle concerns means allowing frequent encounters between individuals in a variant population. Third, there has to be some means of differentially amplifying the number or influence of certain elements in the repertoire that meets the selective criteria. In evolution, the criterion is fitness, in the case of the immune system, it is the tightness of binding between the surface antibodies and the particular foreign molecules, whereas in neuronal systems, value systems (e.g., rewards) are proposed to set criteria to be met by certain neuronal groups whose synapses and circuits, in turn, are selectively amplified. (Note that it is neuronal groups consisting of entire microcircuits with excitatory and inhibitory cellular subtypes that are selected, and not individual neurons.) Together with the further development of such global theories, it will be important to explore, as discussed earlier in the book, how developmental and experiential selection modulate and perhaps differentially amplify certain elements of variant interneuronal populations.

Cajal's Functional Neuroanatomy in the 21st Century

As the previous chapters in this book indicated, there have been significant recent advances especially in three major areas relating to the structural basis of quantitative cortical microcircuit theory. First, the nature of the cellular units has been better defined, through the increasingly precise identification of the individual cellular species that constitute the various cortical networks, leading to the progressively more complete and detailed listing of these diverse cellular constituents. The second major step addressed the thorny problem of synaptic and cellular heterogeneity, encompassing the demonstration of the importance of cell-to-cell variability in distinct, well-defined interneuronal populations, and the quantitative assessment of the number and relative abundance of interneuronal species through the application of the Shannon–Wiener diversity index. The third element related to the key topological principles that underlie network wiring, resulting in the recognition of a surprising order in the architectural design of neuronal networks, and leading to a novel appreciation of the potential role of the inter-areal, long-distance but rarer interneuronal species. These three areas of general advances indicate that we are entering a new, exciting phase in Cajal's paradigm, where the degree of cell-to-cell variability will be treated not as a mere nuisance to be rapidly averaged out, but regarded as an

integral, functionally relevant component of interneuronal heterogeneity in neuronal systems. Thus, the metaphorical cortical crystal
will not break apart just because its constituent cellular elements are
allowed some limited movement in the multidimensional parameter
space, especially if the degree of variance around the mean position
is subjected to strict regulation by various intrinsic and extrinsic
factors.

These three areas of advances will likely deepen our understanding of the computational principles underlying cortical microcircuits
and provide new approaches toward the construction of realistic
models of interneuronal networks. This new phase of research still
draws its inspiration from the revolutionary functional neuroanatomical ideas of Cajal, and it is likely to rely on several additional areas of investigations encorporated by contemporary
neurobiology, including the particularities of interneuronal species
development, the rules of homeostasis and the related molecular
mechanisms regulating the self-tuning of specialized neurons in networks, and on the development of new graph theoretical approaches
that can better capture the essential features of network topologies
specific to cortical circuits. A truly modern functional neuroanatomy
should also be able to eventually determine the genetic and evolutionary basis of interneuronal variability and subtype diversity and
investigate the importance of behaviorally relevant, naturalistic environments in modulating the functional attributes of interneuronal
microcircuits.

Bibliography

Abott, L.F. and LeMasson, G. (1993) Analysis of neuron models with dynamically regulated conductances in model neurons. Neural Computat 5:823–42.

Acsády, L., Arabadzisz, D. and Freund T.F. (1996a) Correlated morphological and neurochemical features identify different subsets of vasoactive intestinal polypeptide-immunoreactive interneurons in rat hippocampus. Neuroscience 73(2):299–315.

Acsády, L., Gorcs, T.J. and Freund, T.F. (1996b) Different populations of vasoactive intestinal polypeptide-immunoreactive interneurons are specialized to control pyramidal cells or interneurons in the hippocampus. Neuroscience 73(2):317–34.

Akbarian, S., Kim, J.J., Potkin, S.G., Hagman, J.O., Tafazzoli, A., Bunney, W.E. Jr and Jones, E.G. (1995) Gene expression for glutamic acid decarboxylase is reduced without loss of neurons in prefrontal cortex of schizophrenics. Arch Gen Psychiatry 52(4):258–66.

Akil, M., Kolachana, B.S., Rothmond, D.A., Hyde, T.M., Weinberger, D.R., and Kleinman, J.E. (2003) Catechol-O-methyltransferase genotype and dopamine regulation in the human brain. J Neurosci 23(6):2008–13.

Albert, R. Jeong, H. and Barabási, A.L. (1999) Internet – Diameter of the World-Wide Web. Nature 401:130–131.

Albert, R., Jeong, H. and Barabási, A.L. (2000) Error and attack tolerance of complex networks. Nature 406:378–82.

Ali, A.B., Bannister, A.P. and Thomson, A.M. (1999) IPSPs elicited in CA1 pyramidal cells by putative basket cells in slices of adult rat hippocampus. Eur J Neurosci 11(5):1741–53.

Amaral, D.G. and Witter, M.P. (1989) The three-dimensional organization of the hippocampal formation: a review of anatomical data. Neuroscience 31(3):571–91.

Andersen, P., Bliss, T.V. and Skrede, K.K. (1971) Lamellar organization of hippocampal pathways. Exp Brain Res 13(2):222–38.

Andersen, P., Soleng, A.F. and Raastad, M. (2000) The hippocampal lamella hypothesis revisited. Brain Res 886(1–2):165–171.

Anderson, K.D. and Reiner, A. (1991) Immunohistochemical localization of DARPP-32 in striatal projection neurons and striatal interneurons: implications for the localization of D1-like dopamine receptors on different types of striatal neurons. Brain Res 568(1–2):235–43.

Anderson, S.A., Eisenstat, D.D., Shi, L. and Rubenstein, J.L. (1997) Interneuron migration from basal forebrain to neocortex: dependence on Dlx genes. Science 278(5337):474–6.

Anderson, S., Mione, M., Yun, K. and Rubenstein, J.L. (1999) Differential origins of neocortical projection and local circuit neurons: role of Dlx genes in neocortical interneuronogenesis. Cereb Cortex 9(6): 646–54.

Anderson, S.A., Marin, O., Horn, C., Jennings, K. and Rubenstein, J.L. (2001) Distinct cortical migrations from the medial and lateral ganglionic eminences. Development 128(3):353–63.

Anderson, S.A., Kaznowski, C.E., Horn, C., Rubenstein, J.L. and McConnell, S.K. (2002) Distinct origins of neocortical projection neurons and interneurons in vivo. Cereb Cortex 12(7):702–9.

Ang, E.S. Jr, Haydar, T.F., Gluncic, V. and Rakic, P. (2003) Four-dimensional migratory coordinates of GABAergic interneurons in the developing mouse cortex. J Neurosci 23(13):5805–15.

Aradi, I. and Soltesz, I. (2002) Modulation of network behaviour by changes in variance in interneuronal properties. J Physiol 538(Pt 1):227–51.

Aradi, I., Santhakumar, V., Chen, K. and Soltesz, I. (2002) Postsynaptic effects of GABAergic synaptic diversity: regulation of neuronal excitability by changes in IPSC variance. Neuropharmacology 43(4): 511–22.

Aradi, I., Santhakumar, V. and Soltesz, I. (2004) Impact of heterogeneous perisomatic IPSC populations on pyramidal cell firing rates. J Neurophysiol 91(6):2849–58.

Arellano, J.I., Munoz, A., Ballesteros-Yanez, I., Sola, R.G. and DeFelipe J. (2004) Histopathology and reorganization of chandelier cells in the human epileptic sclerotic hippocampus. Brain 127(Pt 1):45–64.

Baimbridge, K.G. and Miller, J.J. (1982) Immunohistochemical localization of calcium-binding protein in the cerebellum, hippocampal formation and olfactory bulb of the rat. Brain Res 245(2):223–9.

Baquet, Z.C., Gorski, J.A. and Jones, K.R. (2004) Early striatal dendrite deficits followed by neuron loss with advanced age in the absence of anterograde cortical brain-derived neurotrophic factor. J Neurosci 24(17):4250–8.

Baraban, S.C., Wenzel, H.J., Hochman, D.W. and Schwartzkroin, P.A. (2000) Characterization of heterotopic cell clusters in the hippocampus of rats exposed to methylazoxymethanol in utero. Epilepsy Res 39(2): 87–102.

Barabási, A.L. and Albert, R. (1999) Emergence of scaling in random networks. Science 286(5439):509–12.

Barabási, A.L., Albert, R and Jeong, H. (2000) Scale-free characteristics of random networks: the topology of the World-Wide Web. Physica A 281: 69–77.

Barabási, A.L. (2002) Linked: The New Science of Networks. Cambridge, Mass.: Perseus Publishing.

Barahona, M. and Pecora, L.M. (2002) Synchronization in small-world systems. Phys Rev Lett 89(5):054101.

Bartfeld, E. and Grinvald, A. (1992) Relationships between orientation-preference pinwheels, cytochrome oxidase blobs, and ocular-dominance columns in primate striate cortex. Proc Natl Acad Sci U S A 89(24): 11905–9.

Bartos, M., Vida, I., Frotscher, M., Geiger, J.R. and Jonas P. (2001) Rapid signaling at inhibitory synapses in a dentate gyrus interneuron network. J Neurosci 21(8):2687–98.

Bartos, M., Vida, I., Frotscher, M., Meyer, A., Monyer, H., Geiger, J.R and Jonas, P. (2002) Fast synaptic inhibition promotes synchronized gamma oscillations in hippocampal interneuron networks. Proc Natl Acad Sci U S A 99(20):13222–7.

Beierlein, M., Gibson, J.R. and Connors, B.W. (2000) A network of electrically coupled interneurons drives synchronized inhibition in neocortex. Nat Neurosci 3(9):904–10.

Benes, F.M. and Berretta, S. (2001) GABAergic interneurons: implications for understanding schizophrenia and bipolar disorder. Neuropsychopharmacology 25(1):1–27.

Berghuis, P., Dobszay, M.B., Sousa, K.M., Schulte, G., Mager, P.P., Hartig, W., Gorcs, T.J., Zilberter, Y., Ernfors, P. and Harkany, T. (2004) Brain-derived neurotrophic factor controls functional differentiation and microcircuit formation of selectively isolated fast-spiking GABAergic interneurons. Eur J Neurosci 20(5):1290–306.

Berman, N.J., Douglas, R.J. and Martin, K.A. (1992) GABA-mediated inhibition in the neural networks of visual cortex. Prog Brain Res 90: 443–76.

Bito, H., Deisseroth, K. and Tsien, R.W. (1997) Ca2+-dependent regulation in neuronal gene expression. Curr Opin Neurobiol 7(3):419–29.

Blatow, M., Rozov, A., Katona, I., Hormuzdi, S.G., Meyer, A.H., Whittington, M.A., Caputi, A., Monyer, H. (2003) A novel network of multipolar bursting interneurons generates theta frequency oscillations in neocortex. Neuron 38(5):805–17.

Bolognesi, C., Lando, C., Forni, A., Landini, E., Scarpato, R., Migliore, L., Bonassi, S. (1999) Chromosomal damage and ageing: effect on micronuclei frequency in peripheral blood lymphocytes. Ageing 28(4):393–7.

Bond, J., Roberts, E., Mochida, G.H., Hampshire, D.J., Scott, S., Askham, J.M., Springell, K., Mahadevan, M., Crow, Y.J., Markham, A.F., Walsh, C.A. and Woods, C.G. (2002) ASPM is a major determinant of cerebral cortical size. Nat Genet 32(2):316–20.

Bond, J., Scott, S., Hampshire, D.J., Springell, K., Corry, P., Abramowicz, M.J., Mochida, G.H., Hennekam, R.C., Maher, E.R., Fryns, J..P, Alswaid,

A., Jafri, H., Rashid, Y., Mubaidin, A., Walsh, C.A., Roberts, E. and Woods, C.G. (2003) Protein-truncating mutations in ASPM cause variable reduction in brain size. Am J Hum Genet 73:1170–7.

Braak, H. and Braak, E. (1991) Neuropathological staging of Alzheimer-related changes. Acta Neuropathol (Berl) 82(4):239–59.

Brickley, S.G., Cull-Candy, S.G. and Farrant, M. (1996) Development of a tonic form of synaptic inhibition in rat cerebellar granule cells resulting from persistent activation of GABAA receptors. J Physiol 497(Pt 3):753–9.

Brock, L.G., Coombs, J.S. and Eccles, J.C. (1952) The nature of the monosynaptic excitatory and inhibitory processes in the spinal cord. Proc. R. Soc. London Series B 140: 17–176.

Broadhurst, P.L. (1960) Experiments in psychogenetics: applications of biometrical genetics to the inheritance of behavior. In Experiments in Personality, Vol. 1, Psychogenetics and Psychopharmacology, ed. H.J. Eysenck, pp. 1–102. London: Routledge.

Buchanan, M. (2002) Nexus: Small Worlds and the Groundbreaking Theory of Networks. New York: W.W. Norton & Co.

Bucher, D., Prinz, A.A. and Marder, E. (2005) Animal-to-animal variability in motor pattern production in adults and during growth. J Neurosci 25(7): 1611–1619.

Buckmaster, P.S. and Dudek, F.E. (1999) In vivo intracellular analysis of granule cell axon reorganization in epileptic rats. J Neurophysiol 81(2): 712–21.

Buckmaster, P.S., Zhang, G.F. and Yamawaki, R. (2002) Axon sprouting in a model of temporal lobe epilepsy creates a predominantly excitatory feedback circuit. J Neurosci 22(15):6650–8.

Buettner, V.L., Hill, K.A., Halangoda, A. and Sommer, S.S. (1999) Tandem-base mutations occur in mouse liver and adipose tissue preferentially as G:C to T:A transversions and accumulate with age. Environ Mol Mutagen 33(4):320–4.

Buhl, E.H., Halasy, K. and Somogyi, P. (1994a) Diverse sources of hippocampal unitary inhibitory postsynaptic potentials and the number of synaptic release sites. Nature 368:823–8.

Buhl, E.H., Han, Z.S., Lorinczi, Z., Stezhka, V.V., Karnup, S.V. and Somogyi, P. (1994b) Physiological properties of anatomically identified axo-axonic cells in the rat hippocampus. J Neurophysiol 71(4):1289–307.

Buhl, E.H., Cobb, S.R., Halasy, K. and Somogyi, P. (1995) Properties of unitary IPSPs evoked by anatomically identified basket cells in the rat hippocampus. Eur J Neurosci 7(9):1989–2004.

Bush, P. and Priebe, N. (1998) GABAergic inhibitory control of the transient and sustained components of orientation selectivity in a model micro-column in layer 4 of cat visual cortex. Neural Comput 10(4): 855–67.

Buzsáki, G. (2005) Neuroscience: neurons and navigation. Nature 436(7052): 781–782.

Buzsáki, G., Leung, L.W. and Vanderwolf, C.H. (1983) Cellular bases of hippocampal EEG in the behaving rat. Brain Res 287(2):139–71.

Buzsáki, G., Penttonen, M., Nadasdy, Z. and Bragin, A. (1996) Pattern and inhibition-dependent invasion of pyramidal cell dendrites by fast spikes in the hippocampus in vivo. Proc Natl Acad Sci U S A 93(18):9921–5.

Buzsáki, G., Geisler, C., Henze, D.A. and Wang, X.J. (2004) Interneuron Diversity series: Circuit complexity and axon wiring economy of cortical interneurons. Trends Neurosci 27(4):186–93.

Cajal, S. Ramón y (1888a) Estructura de los centros nerviosos de las aves. Rev. trim. Histol. norm. patol. 1:1–10. (Reprinted in Trabajos escogidos, tomo I. Madrid: Jimenez y Molina. 1924. pp. 305–15.)

Cajal, S. Ramón y (1888b) Estructura del cerebelo. Gac. med. Catalana 11: 449–57.

Cajal, S. Ramón y (1899; 1900) Studies on the human cerebral cortex II. Structure of the motor cortex of man and higher mammals. Revista Trimestral Micrográfica 4:117–200, 1899 and 5:1–11, 1990. English translation in DeFelipe and Jones, 1988.

Cajal, S. Ramón y (orig. 1906; translation: 1967) The structure and connexions of neurons. Nobel Lecture, December 12, 1906. In : Nobel Lectures. Physiology or Medicine 1901–21. New York: Elsevier Publishing Company, pp. 220–53.

Cajal, S. Ramón y (1909, 1911). Histologie du système nerveux de l'homme et des vertébrés (Translation by L. Azoulay). Paris: Maleine, 2 vols.

Cajal, S. Ramón y (1933) ¿ Neuronismo o Reticularismo ? Las pruebas objetivas de la unidad anatómica de las celulas nerviosas. Arch Neurobiol Madrid 13:1–144.

Cajal, S. Ramon y (1954) Neuron theory or reticular theory? Objective evidence of the anatomical unity of nerve cells. Translated from the Spanish original (Cajal, 1933) by Purkiss, M.U. and Fox, C.A. Consejo Superior des Investigaciones Cientificas, Madrid.

Cajal, S. Ramón y (1989) Recollections of My Life. (Translated by E.H. Craigie with the assistance of J.Cano). Philadelphia: American Philosophical Society (1937). Reprinted (1989) Cambridge, Mass.: MIT Press.

Callaway, E.M. (2002) Cell type specificity of local cortical connections. J Neurocytol 31(3–5):231–7.

Cauli, B., Porter, J.T., Tsuzuki, K., Lambolez, B., Rossier, J., Quenet, B. and Audinat, E. (2000) Classification of fusiform neocortical interneurons based on unsupervised clustering. Proc Natl Acad Sci U S A 97(11): 6144–9.

Celio, M.R. (1986) Parvalbumin in most gamma-aminobutyric acid-containing neurons of the rat cerebral cortex. Science 231(4741): 995–997.

Ceranik, K., Bender, R., Geiger, J.R., Monyer, H., Jonas, P., Frotscher, M. and Lubke, J. (1997) A novel type of GABAergic interneuron connecting the input and the output regions of the hippocampus. J Neurosci 17(14):5380–94.

Changizi, M.A. (2003) The Brain from 25,000 feet: High Level Explorations of Brain Complexity, Perception, Induction and Vagueness. New York: Kluwer Academic Press.

Chen, K., Baram, T.Z. and Soltesz, I. (1999) Febrile seizures in the developing brain result in persistent modification of neuronal excitability in limbic circuits. Nat Med 5(8):888–94.

Chen, K., Aradi, I., Thon, N., Eghbal-Ahmadi, M., Baram, T.Z. and Soltesz, I. (2001) Persistently modified h-channels after complex febrile seizures convert the seizure-induced enhancement of inhibition to hyper-excitability. Nat Med 7(3):331–7.

Chen, K., Ratzliff, A., Hilgenberg, L., Gulyás, A., Freund, T.F., Smith, M., Dinh, T.P., Piomelli, D., Mackie, K. and Soltesz, I. (2003) Long-term plasticity of endocannabinoid signaling induced by developmental febrile seizures. Neuron 39(4):599–611.

Chen, Z.Y., Patel, P.D., Sant, G., Meng, C.X., Teng, K.K., Hempstead, B.L. and Lee, F.S. (2004) Variant brain-derived neurotrophic factor (BDNF) (Met66) alters the intracellular trafficking and activity-dependent secretion of wild-type BDNF in neurosecretory cells and cortical neurons. J Neurosci 24(18):4401–11.

Chetsanga, C.J., Tuttle, M., Jacoboni, A. and Johnson, C. (1977) Age-associated structural alterations in senescent mouse brain DNA. Biochim Biophys Acta 474(2):180–7.

Chevassus-au-Louis, N., Baraban, S.C., Gaiarsa, J.L. and Ben-Ari, Y. (1999) Cortical malformations and epilepsy: new insights from animal models. Epilepsia 40(7):811–21.

Chiang, C., Litingtung, Y., Lee, E., Young, K.E., Corden, J.L., Westphal, H. and Beachy, P.A. (1996) Cyclopia and defective axial patterning in mice lacking Sonic hedgehog gene function. Nature 383(6599):407–13.

Chow, A., Erisir, A., Farb, C., Nadal, M.S., Ozaita, A., Lau, D., Welker, E. and Rudy, B. (1999) K(+) channel expression distinguishes subpopulations of parvalbumin- and somatostatin-containing neocortical interneurons. J Neurosci 19(21):9332–45.

Chu, Z., Galarreta, M. and Hestrin, S. (2003) Synaptic interactions of late-spiking neocortical neurons in layer 1. J Neurosci 23(1):96–102.

Clarke, E. and Jacyna, L.S. (1987) Nineteenth-Century Origins of Neuroscientific Concepts. Berkeley and Los Angeles: University of California Press.

Clarke, E. and O'Malley, C.D. (1968) The Human Brain and Spinal Cord. Berkeley: University of California Press.

Cobb, S.R., Buhl, E.H., Halasy, K., Paulsen, O. and Somogyi, P. (1995) Synchronization of neuronal activity in hippocampus by individual GABAergic interneurons. Nature 378:75–8.

Cobos, I., Calcagnotto, M.E., Vilaythong, A.J., Thwin, M.T., Noebels, J.L., Baraban, S.C. and Rubenstein, J.L. (2005) Mice lacking Dlx1 show subtype-specific loss of interneurons, reduced inhibition and epilepsy. Nat Neurosci 8(8):1059–1068.

Colom, L.V. and Bland, B.H. (1987) State-dependent spike train dynamics of hippocampal formation neurons: evidence for theta-on and theta-off cells. Brain Res 422(2):277–86.

Connors,, B.W. and Gutnick, M.J. (1990) Intrinsic firing patterns of diverse neocortical neurons. Trends Neurosci 13(3):99–104.

Coombs, J.S, Eccles, J.C. and Fatt, P. (1955) The specific ionic conductances and the ionic movements across the motoneuronal membrane that produce the inhibitory post-synaptic potential. J Physiol 130(2): 326–74.

Cope, D.W., Maccaferri, G., Marton, L.F., Roberts, J.D., Cobden, P.M. and Somogyi, P. (2002) Cholecystokinin-immunopositive basket and Schaffer collateral-associated interneurones target different domains of pyramidal cells in the CA1 area of the rat hippocampus. Neuroscience 109(1):63–80.

Coskun, P.E., Beal, M.F. and Wallace, D.C. (2004) Alzheimer's brains harbor somatic mtDNA control-region mutations that suppress mitochondrial transcription and replication. Proc Natl Acad Sci U S A 101(29): 10726–31.

Cossart, R., Dinocourt, C., Hirsch, J.C., Merchan-Perez, A., De Felipe, J., Ben-Ari, Y., Esclapez, M. and Bernard, C. (2001) Dendritic but not somatic GABAergic inhibition is decreased in experimental epilepsy. Nat Neurosci 4(1):52–62.

Coulter, D.A. (2001) Epilepsy-associated plasticity in gamma-aminobutyric acid receptor expression, function, and inhibitory synaptic properties. Int Rev Neurobiol 45:237–52.

Csicsvari, J., Hirase, H., Czurko, A., Mamiya, A. and Buzsáki, G. (1999) Oscillatory coupling of hippocampal pyramidal cells and interneurons in the behaving rat. J Neurosci 19(1):274–87.

Curry, J., Karnaoukhova, L., Guenette, G.C. and Glickman, B.W. (1999) Influence of sex, smoking and age on human hprt mutation frequencies and spectra. Genetics 152(3):1065–77.

Darwin, C. (1859) On the Origin of Species by Means of Natural Selection, Or the Preservation of Races in the Struggle for Life. London: J. Murray. (Reprint edition: The Modern Library, New York, 1998).

Dash, P.K., Mach, S.A. and Moore, A.N. (2001) Enhanced neurogenesis in the rodent hippocampus following traumatic brain injury. J Neurosci Res 63(4):313–9.

Dass, S.B., Ali, S.F., Heflich, R.H. and Casciano, D.A. (1977) Frequency of spontaneous and induced micronuclei in the peripheral blood of aging mice. Mutat Res 381(1):105–10.

Davenport, C.J., Brown, W.J. and Babb, T.L. (1990) Sprouting of GABAergic and mossy fiber axons in dentate gyrus following intrahippocampal kainate in the rat. Exp Neurol 109(2):180–90.

Davis, G.W. and Bezprozvanny, I. (2001) Maintaining the stability of neural function: a homeostatic hypothesis. Annu Rev Physiol 63:847–69.

Dayan, P. and Abbott, L.F. (2001) Theoretical Neuroscience. Computational and Mathematical Modeling of Neural Systems. Cambridge, Mass.: MIT Press.

Deacon, T.W., Pakzaban, P. and Isacson, O. (1994) The lateral ganglionic eminence is the origin of cells committed to striatal phenotypes: neural transplantation and developmental evidence. Brain Res 668(1–2): 211–9.

de Boer, J.G. and Glickman, B.W. (1998) The lacI gene as a target for mutation in transgenic rodents and Escherichia coli. Genetics 148(4): 1441–51.

DeFelipe, J. and Jones, E.G. (1988) Cajal on the Cerebral Cortex: An Annotated Translation of the Complete Writings. New York Oxford University Press.

Deller, T., Frotscher, M. and Nitsch, R. (1995) Morphological evidence for the sprouting of inhibitory commissural fibers in response to the lesion of the excitatory entorhinal input to the rat dentate gyrus. J Neurosci 15(10):6868–78.

Denaxa, M., Chan, C.H., Schachner, M., Parnavelas, J.G. and Karagogeos, D. (2001) The adhesion molecule TAG-1 mediates the migration of cortical interneurons from the ganglionic eminence along the corticofugal fiber system. Development 128(22):4635–44.

Desai, N.S., Rutherford, L.C. and Turrigiano, G.G. (1999) Plasticity in the intrinsic excitability of cortical pyramidal neurons. Nat Neurosci 2(6): 515–20.

Devries, S.H. and Baylor, D.A. (1997) Mosaic arrangement of ganglion cell receptive fields in rabbit retina. J Neurophysiol 78(4):2048–60.

Doherty, J. and Dingledine, R. (2001) Reduced excitatory drive onto interneurons in the dentate gyrus after status epilepticus. J Neurosci 21(6):2048–57.

Dolle, M.E., Snyder, W.K., Gossen, J.A., Lohman, P.H. and Vijg, J. (2000) Distinct spectra of somatic mutations accumulated with age in mouse heart and small intestine. Proc Natl Acad Sci U S A 97(15):8403–8.

Douglas, R.J., Martin, K.A.C. and Whitteridge, D. (1989) A canonical microcircuit for neocortex. Neural Computation 1: 480–488.

Douglas, R.J. and Martin, K.A. (1991) A functional microcircuit for cat visual cortex. J Physiol 440:735–69.

Douglas, R.J. and Martin, K.A. (2004) Neuronal circuits of the neocortex. Annu Rev Neurosci. 27:419–51

Driver, C. (2004) What the papers say: where is the somatic mutation that causes aging? Bioessays. 26(11):1160–3.

Dudai, Y. (1988) Neurogenetic dissection of learning and short-term memory in Drosophila. Annu Rev Neurosci 11:537–63.

Dyhrfjeld-Johnsen, J., Santhakumar, V., Huerta, R., Tsimring, L. & Soltesz, I. (2004) Graph structure of neuronal network in the dentate gyrus. 2004 Abstract Viewer/Itinerary Planner. Washington, DC: Society for Neuroscience, Online. Program No. 853.5.

Dyhrfjeld-Johnsen, J. and Soltesz, I. (2004) Dendritic h channelopathy in epileptogenesis. Neuron 44(3):402–3.

Eccles, J.C., Ito, M. and Szentágothai, J. (1967) The Cerebellum as a Neuronal Machine. New York: Springer-Verlag.

Edelman, G.M. (1993) Neural Darwinism: selection and reentrant signaling in higher brain function. Neuron 10(2):115–25.

Edelman, G. (2004) Wider Than the Sky: The Phenomenal Gift of Consciousness. New Haven and London: Yale University Press.

Egan, M.F., Goldberg, T.E., Kolachana, B.S., Callicott, J.H., Mazzanti, C.M., Straub, R.E., Goldman, D. and Weinberger, D.R. (2001) Effect of COMT Val108/158 Met genotype on frontal lobe function and risk for schizophrenia. Proc Natl Acad Sci U S A 98(12):6917–22.

Egan, M.F., Kojima, M., Callicott, J.H., Goldberg, T.E., Kolachana, B.S., Bertolino, A., Zaitsev, E., Gold, B., Goldman, D., Dean, M., Lu, B. and Weinberger, D.R. (2003) The BDNF val66met polymorphism affects activity-dependent secretion of BDNF and human memory and hippocampal function. Cell 112(2):257–69.

Egeland, J.A., Gerhard, D.S., Pauls, D.L., Sussex, J.N., Kidd, K.K., Allen, C.R., Hostetter, A.M. and Housman, D.E. (1987) Bipolar affective disorders linked to DNA markers on chromosome 11. Nature 325(6107):783–7.

Elowitz, M.B., Levine, A.J., Siggia, E.D. and Swain, P.S. (2002) Stochastic gene expression in a single cell. Science 297(5584):1183–6.

Erdös, P. and Rényi, A (1960) On the evolution of random graphs. Publ Math Inst Hung Acad Sci 5:17–61.

Ericson, J., Muhr, J., Placzek, M., Lints, T., Jessell, T.M. and Edlund, T. (1995) Sonic hedgehog induces the differentiation of ventral forebrain neurons: a common signal for ventral patterning within the neural tube. Cell 81(5):747–56.

Ertel, S.I. and Ertel, E.A. (1997) Low-voltage-activated T-type Ca2+ channels. Trends Pharmacol Sci 18(2):37–42.

Evans, P.D., Anderson, J.R., Vallender, E.J., Gilbert. S.L., Malcom, C.M., Dorus, S. and Lahn, B.T. (2004) Adaptive evolution of ASPM, a major determinant of cerebral cortical size in humans. Human Molecular Genetics 13: 489–494.

Farrant, M. and Nusser, Z. (2005) Variations on an inhibitory theme: phasic and tonic activation of GABA(A) receptors. Nat Rev Neurosci 6(3): 215–229.

Fell, D.A. and Wagner, A. (2000) The small world of metabolism. Nat Biotechnol 18(11):1121–2.

Fenech, M. (1998) Chromosomal damage rate, aging, and diet. Ann N Y Acad Sci 854:23–36.

Ferezou, I., Cauli, B., Hill, E.L., Rossier, J., Hamel, E. and Lambolez, B. (2002) 5-HT3 receptors mediate serotonergic fast synaptic excitation of neocortical vasoactive intestinal peptide/cholecystokinin interneurons. J Neurosci 22(17):7389–97.

Ferraguti, F., Cobden, P., Pollard, M., Cope, D., Shigemoto, R., Watanabe, M. and Somogyi, P. (2004) Immunolocalization of metabotropic glutamate receptor 1alpha (mGluR1alpha) in distinct classes of interneuron in the CA1 region of the rat hippocampus. Hippocampus 14(2):193–215.

Figurov, A., Pozzo-Miller, L.D., Olafsson, P., Wang, T. and Lu, B. (1996) Regulation of synaptic responses to high-frequency stimulation and LTP by neurotrophins in the hippocampus. Nature 381(6584):706–9.

Fisahn, A., Pike, F.G., Buhl, E.H. and Paulsen, O. (1998) Cholinergic induction of network oscillations at 40 Hz in the hippocampus in vitro. Nature 394(6689):186–9.

Flames, N., Long, J.E., Garratt, A.N., Fischer, T.M., Gassmann, M., Birchmeier, C., Lai, C., Rubenstein, J.L. and Marin, O. (2004) Short- and long-range attraction of cortical GABAergic interneurons by neuregulin-1. Neuron 44(2):251–61.

Fleck, M.W., Hirotsune, S., Gambello, M.J., Phillips-Tansey, E., Suares, G., Mervis, R.F., Wynshaw-Boris, A. and McBain, C.J. (2000) Hippocampal abnormalities and enhanced excitability in a murine model of human lissencephaly. J Neurosci 20(7):2439–50.

Földy, C., Aradi, I., Howard, A. and Soltesz, I. (2004) Diversity beyond variance: modulation of firing rates and network coherence by GABAergic subpopulations. Eur J Neurosci 19(1):119–30.

Földy, C., Dyhrfjeld-Johnsen, J. and Soltesz, I. (2005) Structure of cortical microcircuit theory. J Physiol 562(Pt 1):47–54.

Frazier, C.J., Rollins, Y.D., Breese, C.R., Leonard, S., Freedman, R. and Dunwiddie, T.V. (1998) Acetylcholine activates an alpha-bungarotoxin-sensitive nicotinic current in rat hippocampal interneurons, but not pyramidal cells. J Neurosci 18(4):1187–95.

Freedman, R., Wetmore, C., Stromberg, I., Leonard, S. and Olson L. (1993) Alpha-bungarotoxin binding to hippocampal interneurons: immunocytochemical characterization and effects on growth factor expression. J Neurosci 13(5):1965–75.

Freund, T.F., Gulyás, A.I., Acsády, L., Gorcs, T. and Toth, K. (1990) Serotonergic control of the hippocampus via local inhibitory interneurons. Proc Natl Acad Sci U S A 87(21):8501–5.

Freund, T.F. and Antal, M. (1988) GABA-containing neurons in the septum control inhibitory interneurons in the hippocampus. Nature 336(6195): 170–3.

Freund, T.F. and Buzsáki, G. (1996) Interneurons of the hippocampus. Hippocampus 6(4):347–470.

Freund, T.F. (2003) Interneuron Diversity series: Rhythm and mood in perisomatic inhibition. Trends Neurosci 26(9):489–95.

Fukuda, T. and Kosaka, T. (2000) Gap junctions linking the dendritic network of GABAergic interneurons in the hippocampus. J Neurosci 20(4): 1519–28.

Galarreta, M. and Hestrin, S. (1999) A network of fast-spiking cells in the neocortex connected by electrical synapses. Nature 402:72–5.

Galarreta, M. and Hestrin, S. (2001) Electrical synapses between GABA-releasing interneurons. Nat Rev Neurosci 2(6):425–33.

Galarreta, M. and Hestrin, S. (2002) Electrical and chemical synapses among parvalbumin fast-spiking GABAergic interneurons in adult mouse neocortex. Proc Natl Acad Sci U S A 99(19):12438–43.

Galarreta, M., Erdelyi, F., Szabo, G., Hestrin, S. (2004) Electrical coupling among irregular-spiking GABAergic interneurons expressing cannabinoid receptors. J Neurosci 24(44):9770–8.

Ganter, P., Szucs, P., Paulsen, O. and Somogyi, P. (2004) Properties of horizontal axo-axonic cells in stratum oriens of the hippocampal CA1 area of rats in vitro. Hippocampus 14(2):232–43.

Gibson, J.R., Beierlein, M. and Connors, B.W. (1999) Two networks of electrically coupled inhibitory neurons in neocortex. Nature 402(6757): 75–9.

Gilbert, C.D. and Wiesel, T.N. (1979) Morphology and intracortical projections of functionally characterised neurones in the cat visual cortex. Nature 280(5718):120–5.

Gilmore, E.C. and Herrup, K. (2001) Neocortical cell migration: GABAergic neurons and cells in layers I and VI move in a cyclin-dependent kinase 5-independent manner. J Neurosci 21(24):9690–700.

Gloveli, T., Dugladze, T., Saha, S., Monyer, H., Heinemann, U., Traub, R.D., Whittington, M.A. and Buhl, E.H. (2005) Differential involvement of oriens/pyramidale interneurones in hippocampal network oscillations in vitro. J Physiol 562(Pt 1):131–47.

Golgi, C. (1873) On the structure of the grey matter of the brain. (Translated by M. Santini). In: Golgi Centennial Symposium (1975, M. Santini, ed.). New York: Raven. pp. 647–50.

Golomb, D. and Rinzel, J. (1993) Dynamics of globally coupled inhibitory neurons with heterogeneity. Phys Rev E Stat Phys Plasmas Fluids Relat Interdiscip Topics 48(6):4810–4814.

Golowasch, J., Goldman, M.S., Abbott, L.F. and Marder, E. (2002) Failure of averaging in the construction of a conductance-based neuron model. J Neurophysiol 87(2):1129–31.

Gorski, J.A., Zeiler, S.R., Tamowski, S. and Jones, K.R. (2003) Brain-derived neurotrophic factor is required for the maintenance of cortical dendrites. J Neurosci 23(17):6856–65.

Gossen, J.A., de Leeuw, W.J., Tan, C.H., Zwarthoff, E.C., Berends, F., Lohman, P.H., Knook, D.L. and Vijg, J. (1989) Efficient rescue of integrated shuttle vectors from transgenic mice: a model for studying mutations in vivo. Proc Natl Acad Sci U S A 86(20):7971–5.

Grastyan, E., Lissak, K., Madarasz, I. And Donhoffer, H. (1959) Hippocampal electrical activity during the development of conditioned reflexes. Electroencephalogr Clin Neurophysiol Suppl 11(3):409–30.

Gray, E.G. (1961) The granule cells, mossy synapses and Purkinje spine synapses of the cerebellum: light and electron microscope observations. J Anat 95:345–56.

Gray, C.M. and McCormick, D.A. (1996) Chattering cells: superficial pyramidal neurons contributing to the generation of synchronous oscillations in the visual cortex. Science 274(5284):109–13.

Guare, J. (1990) Six Degrees of Separation: A Play. New York: Vintage Books.

Gulyás, A.I., Miles, R., Hajos, N. and Freund, T.F. (1993) Precision and variability in postsynaptic target selection of inhibitory cells in the hippocampal CA3 region. Eur J Neurosci 5(12):1729–51.

Gulyás, A.I., Hajos, N. and Freund, T.F. (1996;) Interneurons containing calretinin are specialized to control other interneurons in the rat hippocampus. J Neurosci 16(10):3397–411.

Gulyás, A.I., Toth, K., McBain, C.J. and Freund, T.F. (1998) Stratum radiatum giant cells: a type of principal cell in the rat hippocampus. Eur J Neurosci 10(12):3813–22.

Gulyás, A.I., Megias, M., Emri, Z. and Freund, T.F. (1999) Total number and ratio of excitatory and inhibitory synapses converging onto single interneurons of different types in the CA1 area of the rat hippocampus. J Neurosci 19(22):10082–97.

Gulyás, A.I., Hajos, N., Katona, I. and Freund, T.F. (2003) Interneurons are the local targets of hippocampal inhibitory cells which project to the medial septum. Eur J Neurosci 17(9):1861–72.

Gupta, A., Wang, Y. and Markram, H. (2000) Organizing principles for a diversity of GABAergic interneurons and synapses in the neocortex. Science 287(5451):273–8.

Gutierrez, R. and Heinemann, U. (2001) Kindling induces transient fast inhibition in the dentate gyrus-CA3 projection. Eur J Neurosci 13(7): 1371–9.

Gutierrez R. (2002) Activity-dependent expression of simultaneous glutamatergic and GABAergic neurotransmission from the mossy fibers in vitro. J Neurophysiol 87(5):2562–70.

Guzowski, J.F., McNaughton, B.L., Barnes, C.A. and Worley, P.F. (1999) Environment-specific expression of the immediate-early gene Arc in hippocampal neuronal ensembles. Nat Neurosci 2(12):1120–4.

Hafting, T., Fyhn, M., Molden, S., Moser, M.B. and Moser, E.I. (2005) Microstructure of a spatial map in the entorhinal cortex. Nature 436(7052):801–806.

Hajos, N. and Mody. I. (1997) Synaptic communication among hippocampal interneurons: properties of spontaneous IPSCs in morphologically identified cells. J Neurosci 17(21):8427–42.

Hajos, N., Papp, E.C., Acsády, L., Levey, A.I. and Freund, T.F. (1998) Distinct interneuron types express m2 muscarinic receptor immunoreactivity on their dendrites or axon terminals in the hippocampus. Neuroscience 82(2):355–76.

Hajos, N., Palhalmi, J., Mann, E.O., Nemeth, B., Paulsen, O. and Freund, T.F. (2004) Spike timing of distinct types of GABAergic interneuron during hippocampal gamma oscillations in vitro. J Neurosci 24(41): 9127–37.

Halasy, K. and Somogyi, P. (1993) Subdivisions in the multiple GABAergic innervation of granule cells in the dentate gyrus of the rat hippocampus. Eur J Neurosci 5(5):411–29.

Halasy, K., Buhl, E.H., Lorinczi, Z., Tamas, G. and Somogyi, P. (1996) Synaptic target selectivity and input of GABAergic basket and bistratified interneurons in the CA1 area of the rat hippocampus. Hippocampus 6(3):306–29.

Hamasaki, T., Goto, S., Nishikawa, S. and Ushio, Y. (2001) A role of netrin-1 in the formation of the subcortical structure striatum: repulsive action on the migration of late-born striatal neurons. J Neurosci 21(12): 4272–80.

Han, Z.S., Buhl, E.H., Lorinczi, Z., Somogyi, P. (1993) A high degree of spatial selectivity in the axonal and dendritic domains of physiologically identified local-circuit neurons in the dentate gyrus of the rat hippocampus. Eur J Neurosci 5(5):395–410.

Hariri, A.R., Goldberg, T.E., Mattay, V.S., Kolachana, B.S., Callicott, J.H., Egan, M.F. and Weinberger, D.R. (2003) Brain-derived neurotrophic factor val66met polymorphism affects human memory-related hippocampal activity and predicts memory performance. J Neurosci 23(17):6690–4.

Harris, K.M., Marshall, P.E. and Landis, D.M. (1985) Ultrastructural study of cholecystokinin-immunoreactive cells and processes in area CA1 of the rat hippocampus. J Comp Neurol 233(2):147–58.

Heinz, A., Braus, D.F., Smolka, M.N., Wrase, J., Puls, I., Hermann, D., Klein, S., Grusser, S.M., Flor, H., Schumann, G., Mann, K. and Buchel, C. (2005) Amygdala-prefrontal coupling depends on a genetic variation of the serotonin transporter. Nat Neurosci 8(1):20–1.

Hestrin, S. and Armstrong, W.E. (1996) Morphology and physiology of cortical neurons in layer I. J Neurosci 16: 5290–5300.

Hevers, W. and Luddens, H. (1998) The diversity of GABAA receptors. Pharmacological and electrophysiological properties of GABAA channel subtypes. Mol Neurobiol 18(1):35–86.

Hill, K.A., Buettner, V.L., Glickman, B.W. and Sommer, S.S. (1999) Spontaneous mutations in the Big Blue transgenic system are primarily mouse derived. Mutat Res 436(1):11–9.

Hill, K.A., Buettner, V.L., Halangoda, A., Kunishige, M., Moore, S.R., Longmate, J., Scaringe, W.A. and Sommer, S.S. (2004) Spontaneous mutation in Big Blue mice from fetus to old age: tissue-specific time courses of mutation frequency but similar mutation types. Environ Mol Mutagen 43(2):110–20.

Hill, S.L. and Tononi, G. (2005) Modeling Sleep and Wakefulness in the Thalamocortical System. J Neurophysiol 93: 1671–1698.

Hirsch, J.C., Agassandian, C., Merchan-Perez, A., Ben-Ari, Y., DeFelipe, J., Esclapez, M. and Bernard, C. (1999) Deficit of quantal release of GABA in experimental models of temporal lobe epilepsy. Nat Neurosci 2(6):499–500.

Hoffmann, A.A. (1994) Behaviour genetics and evolution. In: Slater, P.J.B. and Halliday, T.R., eds., Behavior and Evolution, pp. 7–43. Cambridge: Cambridge University Press.

Houser, C.R. and Esclapez, M. (2003) Downregulation of the alpha5 subunit of the GABA(A) receptor in the pilocarpine model of temporal lobe epilepsy. Hippocampus 13(5):633–45.

Howard, A., Tamas, G. and Soltesz, I. (2005) Lighting the chandelier: New vistas for axo-axonic cells. Trends in Neurosciences 28(6): 310–316.

Hua, J.Y. and Smith, S.J. (2004) Neural activity and the dynamics of central nervous system development. Nat Neurosci 7(4):327–32.

Huang, Z.J., Kirkwood, A., Pizzorusso, T., Porciatti, V., Morales, B., Bear, M.F., Maffei, L. and Tonegawa, S. (1999) BDNF regulates the maturation of inhibition and the critical period of plasticity in mouse visual cortex. Cell 98(6):739–55.

Ischiropoulos, H., Zhu, L. and Beckman, J.S. (1992) Peroxynitrite formation from macrophage-derived nitric oxide. Arch Biochem Biophys 298(2): 446–51.

Jacobson, M. (1993) Foundations of Neuroscience. New York: Plenum Press.

Jeanmonod, D., Rice, F.L. and Van der Loos, H. (1981) Mouse somatosensory cortex: alterations in the barrelfield following receptor injury at different early postnatal ages. Neuroscience 6(8):1503–35.

Jeong, H., Tombor, B., Albert, R., Oltvai, Z.N. and Barabási, A.L. (2000) The large-scale organization of metabolic networks. Nature 407(6804):651–4.

Jeong, H., Mason, S.P., Barabási, A.L. and Oltvai, Z.N. (2001) Lethality and centrality in protein networks. Nature 411(6833):41–2.

Jinno, S. and Kosaka, T. (2002) Immunocytochemical characterization of hippocamposeptal projecting GABAergic nonprincipal neurons in the mouse brain: a retrograde labeling study. Brain Res 945(2):219–31.

Jones, E.G. (1975) Varieties and distribution of non-pyramidal cells in the somatic sensory cortex of the squirrel monkey. J Comp Neurol 160: 205–267.

Jones, E.G. (1993) GABAergic neurons and their role in cortical plasticity in primates. Cereb Cortex. 3(5):361–72.

Jones, E.G. (1999) Colgi, Cajal and the neuron doctrine. J Hist Neurosci 8(2):170–8.

Jones, E.G., Woods, T.M. and Manger, P.R. (2002) Adaptive responses of monkey somatosensory cortex to peripheral and central deafferentation. Neuroscience 111(4):775–97.

Kamme, F., Salunga, R., Yu, J., Tran, D.T., Zhu, J., Luo, L., Bittner, A., Guo, H.Q., Miller, N., Wan, J. and Erlander, M. (2003) Single-cell microarray analysis in hippocampus CA1: demonstration and validation of cellular heterogeneity. J Neurosci 23(9):3607–15.

Kamondi, A., Acsády, L., Wang, X.J. and Buzsáki, G. (1998) Theta oscillations in somata and dendrites of hippocampal pyramidal cells in vivo:activity-dependent phase-precession of action potentials. Hippocampus 8(3):244–261.

Katona, I., Acsády, L., Freund, T.F. (1999a) Postsynaptic targets of somatostatin-immunoreactive interneurons in the rat hippocampus. Neuroscience 88(1):37–55.

Katona, I., Sperlagh, B., Sik, A., Kafalvi, A., Vizi, E.S., Mackie, K. and Freund, T.F. (1999b) Presynaptically located CB1 cannabinoid receptors regulate GABA release from axon terminals of specific hippocampal interneurons. J Neurosci 19(11):4544–58.

Katsumaru, H., Kosaka, T., Heizmann, C.W. and Hama, K. (1988) Gap junctions on GABAergic neurons containing the calcium-binding protein parvalbumin in the rat hippocampus (CA1 region). Exp Brain Res 72(2):363–70.

Kawaguchi, Y. and Kubota, Y. (1997) GABAergic cell subtypes and their synaptic connections in rat frontal cortex. Cereb Cortex 7:476–486.

Khazipov, R., Congar, P. and Ben-Ari, Y. (1995) Hippocampal CA1 lacunosum-moleculare interneurons: modulation of monosynaptic GABAergic IPSCs by presynaptic GABAB receptors. J Neurophysiol 74(5):2126–37.

Kilman, V., van Rossum, M.C. and Turrigiano, G.G. (2002) Activity deprivation reduces miniature IPSC amplitude by decreasing the number of postsynaptic GABA(A) receptors clustered at neocortical synapses. J Neurosci 22(4):1328–37.

Kisvárday, Z.F., Gulyas, A., Beroukas, D., North, J.B., Chubb, I.W. and Somogyi, P. (1990) Synapses, axonal and dendritic patterns of GABA-immunoreactive neurons in human cerebral cortex. Brain 113: 793–812.

Kisvárday, Z.F., Martin, K.A., Whitteridge, D. and Somogyi, P. (1985) Synaptic connections of intracellularly filled clutch cells: a type of small basket cell in the visual cortex of the cat. J Comp Neurol 241(2): 111–37.

Klausberger, T., Roberts, J.D. and Somogyi, P. (2002) Cell type- and input-specific differences in the number and subtypes of synaptic GABA(A) receptors in the hippocampus. J Neurosci 22(7):2513–21.

Klausberger, T., Magill, P.J., Marton, L.F., Roberts, J.D., Cobden, P.M., Buzsáki, G. and Somogyi, P. (2003) Brain-state- and cell-type-specific firing of hippocampal interneurons in vivo. Nature 421(6925):844–8.

Klausberger, T., Marton, L.F., Baude, A., Roberts, J.D., Magill, P.J. and Somogyi, P. (2004) Spike timing of dendrite-targeting bistratified cells during hippocampal network oscillations in vivo. Nat Neurosci 7(1): 41–7.

Knott, G.W., Quairiaux, C., Genoud, C. and Welker, E. (2002) Formation of dendritic spines with GABAergic synapses induced by whisker stimulation in adult mice. Neuron 34(2):265–73.

Kodama, T., Mushiake, H., Shima, K., Nakahama, H. and Yamamoto, M. (1989) Slow fluctuations of single unit activities of hippocampal and thalamic neurons in cats. I. Relation to natural sleep and alert states. Brain Res 487(1):26–34.

Kohler, S.W., Provost, G.S., Fieck, A., Kretz, P.L., Bullock, W.O., Putman, D.L. and Sorge, J.A. and Short, J.M. (1991) Analysis of spontaneous and induced mutations in transgenic mice using a lambda ZAP/lacI shuttle vector. Environ Mol Mutagen 18(4):316–21.

Kohtz, J.D., Baker, D.P., Corte, G. and Fishell, G. (1998) Regionalization within the mammalian telencephalon is mediated by changes in responsiveness to Sonic Hedgehog. Development 125(24):5079–89.

Kölliker, A. (1986) Handbuch der Gewebelehre des Menschen, 6ʰ ed., Vol. 2: Nervensystems des Menschen und der Thiere. Leipzig: Engelmann. [The translation of the passage from this article quoted at the beginning of chapter 2 was from Shepherd, 1991].

Kong, J.H., Fish, D.R., Rockhill, R.L. and Masland, R.H. (2005) Diversity of ganglion cells in the mouse retina: Unsupervised morphological classification and its limits. J Comp Neurol 489(3):293–310.

Kouprina, N., Pavlicek, A., Mochida, G.H., Solomon, G., Gersch, W., Yoon, Y.H., Collura, R., Ruvolo, M., Barrett, J.C., Woods, C.G., Walsh, C.A., Jurka, J. and Larionov, V. (2004) Accelerated evolution of the ASPM gene controlling brain size begins prior to human brain expansion. PLoS Biology 2:E126

Kovalenko, S.A., Kopsidas, G., Kelso, J., Rosenfeldt, F. and Linnane, A.W. (1998) Tissue-specific distribution of multiple mitochondrial DNA rearrangements during human aging. Ann N Y Acad Sci 854:171–81.

Kozloski, J., Hamzei-Sichani, F. and Yuste, R. (2001) Stereotyped position of local synaptic targets in neocortex. Science 293(5531):868–72.

Kuhn, T.S. (1996) The Structure of Scientific Revolutions. Chicago: The University of Chicago Press.

Lacaille, J.C. and Schwartzkroin, P.A. (1988) Stratum lacunosum-moleculare interneurons of hippocampal CA1 region. II. Intrasomatic and intradendritic recordings of local circuit synaptic interactions. J Neurosci 8(4):1411–24.

Lago-Fernandez, L.F., Huerta, R., Corbacho, F. and Siguenza, J.A. (2000)

Fast response and temporal coherent oscillations in small-world networks. Phys Rev Lett 84(12):2758–61.

Lamas, M., Gomez-Lira, G. and Gutierrez, R. (2001) Vesicular GABA transporter mRNA expression in the dentate gyrus and in mossy fiber synaptosomes. Brain Res 93(2):209–14.

Lee, J.L., Everitt, B.J. and Thomas, K.L. (2004) Independent cellular processes for hippocampal memory consolidation and reconsolidation. Science 304(5672):839–43.

Lehmann, H., Ebert, U. and Loscher, W. (1996) Immunocytochemical localization of GABA immunoreactivity in dentate granule cells of normal and kindled rats. Neurosci Lett 212(1):41–4.

LeMasson, G., Marder, E. and Abbott, L.F. (1993) Activity-dependent regulation of conductances in model neurons. Science 259(5103): 1915–7.

Leslie, K.R., Nelson, S.B. and Turrigiano, G.G. (2001) Postsynaptic depolarization scales quantal amplitude in cortical pyramidal neurons. J Neurosci 21(19):RC170.

Letinic, K., Zoncu, R. and Rakic, P. (2002) Origin of GABAergic neurons in the human neocortex. Nature 417(6889):645–9.

Li, C. and Chen, G. (2003) Stability of a neural network model with small-world connections. Phys Rev E Stat Nonlin Soft Matter Phys 68(5 Pt 1):052901.

Li, X.G., Somogyi, P., Tepper, J.M. and Buzsáki, G. (1992) Axonal and dendritic arborization of an intracellularly labeled chandelier cell in the CA1 region of rat hippocampus. Exp Brain Res 90(3):519–25.

Liu, S., Wang, J., Zhu, D., Fu, Y., Lukowiak, K. and Lu, Y.M. (2003) Generation of functional inhibitory neurons in the adult rat hippocampus. J Neurosci 23(3):732–6.

Loreau, M., Naeem, S., Inchausti, P., Bengtsson, J., Grime, J.P., Hector, A., Hooper, D.U., Huston, M.A., Raffaelli, D., Schmid, B., Tilman, D. and Wardle, D.A. (2001) Biodiversity and ecosystem functioning: current knowledge and future challenges. Science 294(5543):804–8.

Losonczy, A., Biro, A.A. and Nusser, Z. (2004) Persistently active cannabinoid receptors mute a subpopulation of hippocampal interneurons. Proc Natl Acad Sci U S A 101(5):1362–7.

Low, K., Crestani, F., Keist, R., Benke, D., Brunig, I., Benson, J.A., Fritschy, J.M., Rulicke, T., Bluethmann, H., Mohler, H. and Rudolph, U. (2000) Molecular and neuronal substrate for the selective attenuation of anxiety. Science 290(5489):131–4.

Lu, T., Pan, Y., Kao, S.Y., Li, C., Kohane, I., Chan, J. and Yankner, B.A. (2004) Gene regulation and DNA damage in the ageing human brain. Nature 429:883–91.

Lytton, W.W. and Sejnowski, T.J. (1991) Simulations of cortical pyramidal neurons synchronized by inhibitory interneurons. J Neurophysiol 66(3):1059–79.

Maccaferri, G. and McBain, C.J. (1996) Long-term potentiation in distinct subtypes of hippocampal nonpyramidal neurons. J Neurosci 16(17): 5334–43.

Maccaferri, G., Toth, K. and McBain, C.J. (1998) Target-specific expression of presynaptic mossy fiber plasticity. Science 279(5355):1368–70.

Maccaferri, G., Roberts, J.D., Szucs, P., Cottingham, C.A., Somogyi, P. (2000) Cell surface domain specific postsynaptic currents evoked by identified GABAergic neurones in rat hippocampus in vitro. J Physiol 524 Pt 1:91–116.

Mackler, S.A., Brooks, B.P. and Eberwine, J.H. (1992) Stimulus-induced coordinate changes in mRNA abundance in single postsynaptic hippocampal CA1 neurons. Neuron 9(3):539–48.

MacNeil, M.A. and Masland, R.H. (1998) Extreme diversity among amacrine cells: implications for function. Neuron 20(5):971–82.

Madach, I. (1862) The Tragedy of Man. (Translated by T.R. Mark, 1989.) New York: Columbia University Press.

Marder, E. and Prinz, A.A. (2002) Modeling stability in neuron and network function: the role of activity in homeostasis. Bioessays 24(12):1145–54.

Markakis, E.A. and Gage, F.H. (1999) Adult-generated neurons in the dentate gyrus send axonal projections to field CA3 and are surrounded by synaptic vesicles. J Comp Neurol 406(4):449–60.

Markram, H., Toledo-Rodriguez, M., Wang, Y., Gupta, A., Silberberg, G. and Wu, C. (2004) Interneurons of the neocortical inhibitory system. Nat Rev Neurosci 5(10):793–807.

Marin, O., Plump, A.S., Flames, N., Sanchez-Camacho, C., Tessier-Lavigne, M. and Rubenstein, J.L. (2003) Directional guidance of interneuron migration to the cerebral cortex relies on subcortical Slit1/2-independent repulsion and cortical attraction. Development 130(9):1889–1901.

Marin, O., Yaron, A., Bagri, A., Tessier-Lavigne, M. and Rubenstein, J.L. (2001) Sorting of striatal and cortical interneurons regulated by semaphorin-neuropilin interactions. Science 293(5531):872–5.

Marin, O. and Rubenstein, J.L. (2003) Cell migration in the forebrain. Annu Rev Neurosci 26:441–83.

Martina, M., Schultz, J.H., Ehmke, H., Monyer, H. and Jonas, P. (1998) Functional and molecular differences between voltage-gated K+ channels of fast-spiking interneurons and pyramidal neurons of rat hippocampus. J Neurosci 18(20):8111–25.

Masland, R.H. (2001) Neuronal diversity in the retina. Curr Opin Neurobiol 11(4):431–6.

Masuda, N. and Aihara, K. (2004) Global and local synchrony of coupled neurons in small-world networks. Biol Cybern 90(4):302–9.

Mathern, G.W., Bertram, E.H. 3rd, Babb, T.L., Pretorius, J.K., Kuhlman, P.A., Spradlin, S. and Mendoza, D. (1997) In contrast to kindled seizures, the frequency of spontaneous epilepsy in the limbic status model correlates with greater aberrant fascia dentate excitatory and inhibitory axon sprouting, and increased staining for N-methyl-D-aspartate, AMPA and GABA(A) receptors. Neuroscience 1997 77(4):1003–19.

Matyas, F., Freund, T.F. and Gulyás, A.I. (2004) Convergence of excitatory and inhibitory inputs onto CCK-containing basket cells in the CA1 area of the rat hippocampus. Eur J Neurosci 19(5):1243–56.

Mayr, E. (1942) Systematics and the Origin of Species. New York: Columbia University Press.

Mayr, E. (1982) The Growth of Biological Thought. Cambridge, Mass.: Belknap Press of Harvard University Press.

McBain, C.J. and Fisahn, A. (2001) Interneurons unbound. Nat Rev Neurosci 2(1):11–23.

McBain, C.J., DiChiara, T.J. and Kauer, J.A. (1994) Activation of metabotropic glutamate receptors differentially affects two classes of hippocampal interneurons and potentiates excitatory synaptic transmission. J Neurosci 14(7):4433–45.

McQuiston, A.R. and Madison, D.V. (1999) Muscarinic receptor activity has multiple effects on the resting membrane potentials of CA1 hippocampal interneurons. J Neurosci 19(14):5693–702.

Metin, C., Denizot, J.P. and Ropert, N. (2000) Intermediate zone cells express calcium-permeable AMPA receptors and establish close contact with growing axons. J Neurosci 20(2):696–708.

Meyer, A.H., van Hooft, J.A. and Monyer, H. (2002) An electrically coupled hippocampal network of cholecystokinin (CCK)-positive GABAergic interneurons revealed by transgenic mice expressing green fluorescent protein in CCK-positive neurons. 2002 Abstract Viewer and Itinerary Planner, Society for Neuroscience, Online. Program No. 936.2.

Meyer, G., Soria, J.M., Martinez-Galan, J.R., Martin-Clemente, B. and Fairen, A. (1998) Different origins and developmental histories of transient neurons in the marginal zone of the fetal and neonatal rat cortex. J Comp Neurol 397(4):493–518.

Micheva, K.D. and Beaulieu, C. (1997) Development and plasticity of the inhibitory neocortical circuitry with an emphasis on the rodent barrel field cortex: a review. Can J Physiol Pharmacol 75(5):470–8.

Miles, R., Toth, K., Gulyás, A.I., Hajos, N. and Freund, T.F. (1996) Differences between somatic and dendritic inhibition in the hippocampus. Neuron 16(4):815–23.

Milgram, S. (1967) The small-world problem. Psychol. Today 2:60–67.

Mizumori, S.J., Barnes, C.A. and McNaughton, B.L. (1990) Behavioral correlates of theta-on and theta-off cells recorded from hippocampal formation of mature young and aged rats. Exp Brain Res 80(2): 365–73.

Mody, I. (2002) The GAD-given right of dentate gyrus granule cells to become GABAergic. Epilepsy Curr 2(5):143–145.

Mody, I. and Pearce, R.A. (2004) Diversity of inhibitory neurotransmission through GABA(A) receptors. Trends Neurosci 27(9):569–75.

Mody, I. (2005) Aspects of the homeostaic plasticity of GABAA receptor-mediated inhibition. J Physiol 562(Pt 1):37–46.

Morales, M. and Bloom, F.E. (1997) The 5-HT3 receptor is present in different subpopulations of GABAergic neurons in the rat telencephalon. J Neurosci 17(9):3157–67.

Moser, E.I. (1996) Altered inhibition of dentate granule cells during spatial learning in an exploration task. J Neurosci 16(3):1247–59.

Mott, D.D. and Dingledine, R. (2003) Interneuron Diversity series: Interneuron research—challenges and strategies. Trends Neurosci 26(9):484–8.

Mountcastle, V.B. (1997) The columnar organization of the neocortex. Brain 120 (Pt 4):701–22.

Mukherjee, A.B. and Thomas, S. (1997) A longitudinal study of human age-related chromosomal analysis in skin fibroblasts. Exp Cell Res 235(1):161–9.

Nelson, S. (2002) Cortical microcircuits: diverse or canonical? Neuron 36(1):19–27.

Netoff, T.I., Clewley, R., Arno, S., Keck, T. and White, J.A. (2004) Epilepsy in small-world networks. J Neurosci 24(37):8075–83.

Newman, M.E. (2001) Clustering and preferential attachment in growing networks. Phys Rev E Stat Nonlin Soft Matter Phys 64(2 Pt 2):025102.

Nick, T.A. and Ribera, A.B. (2000) Synaptic activity modulates presynaptic excitability. Nat Neurosci 3(2):142–9.

Nicoll, R.A. (1994) Neuroscience. Cajal's rational psychology. Nature 368 (6474):808–9.

Nitsch, R. and Frotscher, M. (1992) Reduction of posttraumatic trans-neuronal "early gene" activation and dendritic atrophy by the N-methyl-D-aspartate receptor antagonist MK-801. Proc Natl Acad Sci U S A 89(11):5197–200.

Nitz, D. and McNaughton, B. (2004) Differential modulation of CA1 and dentate gyrus interneurons during exploration of novel environments. J Neurophysiol 91(2):863–72.

Nunzi, M.G., Gorio, A., Milan, F., Freund, T.F., Somogyi, P. and Smith, A.D. (1985) Cholecystokinin-immunoreactive cells form symmetrical synaptic contacts with pyramidal and nonpyramidal neurons in the hippocampus. J Comp Neurol 237(4):485–505.

Nusser, Z., Sieghart, W., Stephenson, F.A. and Somogyi, P. (1996) The alpha 6 subunit of the GABAA receptor is concentrated in both inhibitory and excitatory synapses on cerebellar granule cells. J Neurosci 16(1): 103–14.

Nyiri, G., Freund, T.F. and Somogyi, P. (2001) Input-dependent synaptic targeting of alpha(2)-subunit-containing GABA(A) receptors in synapses of hippocampal pyramidal cells of the rat. Eur J Neurosci 13(3):428–42.

Nyiri, G., Stephenson, F.A., Freund, T.F. and Somogyi, P. (2003) Large variability in synaptic N-methyl-D-aspartate receptor density on interneurons and a comparison with pyramidal-cell spines in the rat hippocampus. Neuroscience 119(2):347–63.

Ono, T., Miyamura, Y., Ikehata, H., Yamanaka, H., Kurishita, A., Yamamoto, K., Suzuki, T., Nohmi, T., Hayashi, M. and Sofuni, T. (1995) Spontaneous mutant frequency of lacZ gene in spleen of transgenic mouse increases with age. Mutat Res 338(1–6):183–8.

Ono, T., Ikehata, H., Nakamura, S., Saito, Y., Hosoi, Y., Takai, Y., Yamada, S., Onodera, J. and Yamamoto, K. (2000) Age-associated increase of spontaneous mutant frequency and molecular nature of mutation in newborn and old lacZ-transgenic mouse. Mutat Res 447(2):165–77.

Palade, G.E. and Palay, S.L. (1954) Electron microscope observations of interneuronal and neuromuscular synapses. Anat Rec. 118: 335–336.

Papp, E.C., Hajos, N., Acsády, L. and Freund, T.F. (1999) Medial septal and median raphe innervation of vasoactive intestinal polypeptide-containing interneurons in the hippocampus. Neuroscience 90(2):369–82.

Paradis, S., Sweeney, S.T. and Davis, G.W. (2001) Homeostatic control of presynaptic release is triggered by postsynaptic membrane depolarization. Neuron 30(3):737–49.

Parent, J.M., Yu, T.W., Leibowitz, R.T., Geschwind, D.H., Sloviter, R.S. and Lowenstein, D.H. (1997) Dentate granule cell neurogenesis is increased by seizures and contributes to aberrant network reorganization in the adult rat hippocampus. J Neurosci 17(10):3727–38.

Parra, P., Gulyás, A.I. and Miles, R. (1998) How many subtypes of inhibitory cells in the hippocampus? Neuron 20(5):983–93.

Pawelzik, H., Bannister, A.P., Deuchars, J., Ilia, M. and Thomson, A.M. (1999) Modulation of bistratified cell IPSPs and basket cell IPSPs by pentobarbitone sodium, diazepam and Zn2+: dual recordings in slices of adult rat hippocampus. Eur J Neurosci 11(10):3552–64.

Pawelzik, H., Hughes, D.I. and Thomson, A.M. (2002) Physiological and morphological diversity of immunocytochemically defined parvalbu- min- and cholecystokinin-positive interneurones in CA1 of the adult rat hippocampus. J Comp Neurol 443(4):346–67.

Pawelzik, H., Hughes, D.I. and Thomson, A.M. (2003) Modulation of inhibitory autapses and synapses on rat CA1 interneurones by GABA(A) receptor ligands. J Physiol 546(Pt 3):701–16.

Pearce, B.D., Steffensen, S.C., Paoletti, A.D., Henriksen, S.J. and Buchmeier, M.J. (1996) Persistent dentate granule cell hyperexcitability after neonatal infection with lymphocytic choriomeningitis virus. J Neurosci 16(1):220–8.

Peters, A., Proskauer, C.C. and Ribak, C.E. (1982) Chandelier cells in rat visual cortex. J Comp Neurol 206(4):397–416.

Pezawas, L., Verchinski, B.A., Mattay, V.S., Callicott, J.H., Kolachana, B.S., Straub, R.E., Egan, M.F., Meyer-Lindenberg, A. and Weinberger, D.R.

(2004) The brain-derived neurotrophic factor val66met polymorphism
and variation in human cortical morphology. J Neurosci 24(45):
10099–102.

Pike, F.G., Goddard, R.S., Suckling, J.M., Ganter, P., Kasthuri, N. and
Paulsen, O. (2000) Distinct frequency preferences of different types of
rat hippocampal neurones in response to oscillatory input currents. J
Physiol 529(Pt 1):205–13.

Pineault, D. (1994) Golgi-like labeling of a single neuron recorded
extracellularly. Neurosci Lett 170(2):255–60.

Pleasure, S.J., Anderson, S., Hevner, R., Bagri, A., Marin, O., Lowenstein,
D.H. and Rubenstein, J.L. (2000) Cell migration from the ganglionic
eminences is required for the development of hippocampal GABAergic
interneurons. Neuron 28(3):727–40.

Poisbeau, P., Williams, S.R. and Mody, I. (1997) Silent GABAA synapses
during flurazepam withdrawal are region-specific in the hippocampal
formation. J Neurosci 17(10):3467–75.

Polleux, F., Whitford, K.L., Dijkhuizen, P.A., Vitalis, T. and Ghosh, A. (2002)
Control of cortical interneuron migration by neurotrophins and PI3-
kinase signaling. Development 129(13):3147–60.

Polley, D.B., Kvasnak, E. and Frostig, R.D. (2004) Naturalistic experience
transforms sensory maps in the adult cortex of caged animals. Nature
429(6987):67–71.

Pouille, F. and Scanziani, M. (2004) Routing of spike series by dynamic
circuits in the hippocampus. Nature 429(6993):717–23.

Powell, E.M., Mars, W.M. and Levitt, P. (2001) Hepatocyte growth factor/
scatter factor is a motogen for interneurons migrating from the ventral
to dorsal telencephalon. Neuron 30(1):79–89.

Price, C.J., Cauli, B., Kovacs, E.R., Kulik, A., Lambolez, B., Shigemoto, R.
and Capogna M. (2005) Neurogliaform neurons form a novel inhibitory
network in the hippocampal CAI area. J Neurosci 25(29):6775–6786.

Prince, D.A. and Jacobs, K. (1998) Inhibitory function in two models of
chronic epileptogenesis. Epilepsy Res 32(1–2):83–92.

Prinz, A.A., Bucher, D. and Marder, E. (2004) Similar network activity from
disparate circuit parameters. Nat Neurosci 7(12):1345–1352.

Rakic, P. (1972) Mode of cell migration to the superficial layers of fetal
monkey neocortex. J Comp Neurol 145(1):61–83.

Rakic, P. (1988) Specification of cerebral cortical areas. Science 241
(4862):170–6.

Rakic, S. and Zecevic, N. (2003) Emerging complexity of layer I in human
cerebral cortex. Cereb Cortex 13(10):1072–83.

Ramirez, M. and Gutierrez, R. (2001) Activity-dependent expression of
GAD67 in the granule cells of the rat hippocampus. Brain Res 917
(2):139–46.

Raper, J.A. (2000) Semaphorins and their receptors in vertebrates and
invertebrates. Curr Opin Neurobiol 10(1):88–94.

Ratzliff, A.D. and Soltesz, I. (2000) Differential expression of cytoskeletal proteins in the dendrites of parvalbumin-positive interneurons versus granule cells in the adult rat dentate gyrus. Hippocampus 10(2): 162–8.

Ratzliff, A.D. and Soltesz, I. (2001) Differential immunoreactivity for alpha-actinin-2, an N-methyl-D-aspartate-receptor/actin binding protein, in hippocampal interneurons. Neuroscience 103(2):337–49.

Robinson, D.R., Goodall, K., Albertini, R.J., O'Neill, J.P., Finette, B., Sala-Trepat, M., Moustacchi, E., Tates, A.D., Beare, D.M., Green MH, et al. (1994) An analysis of in vivo hprt mutant frequency in circulating T-lymphocytes in the normal human population: a comparison of four datasets. Mutat Res 313(2–3):227–47.

Romo-Parra, H., Vivar, C., Maqueda, J., Morales, M.A. and Gutierrez, R. (2003) Activity-dependent induction of multitransmitter signaling onto pyramidal cells and interneurons of hippocampal area CA3. J Neurophysiol 89(6):3155–67.

Ross, S.T. and Soltesz, I. (2000) Selective depolarization of interneurons in the early posttraumatic dentate gyrus: involvement of the Na(+)/K(+)-ATPase. J Neurophysiol 83(5):2916–30.

Ross, S.T. and Soltesz, I. (2001) Long-term plasticity in interneurons of the dentate gyrus. Proc Natl Acad Sci U S A 98(15):8874–9.

Ross, W.N. (1989) Changes in intracellular calcium during neuron activity. Annu Rev Physiol 51:491–506.

Rudy, B. and McBain, C.J. (2001) Kv3 channels: voltage-gated K+ channels designed for high-frequency repetitive firing. Trends Neurosci 24(9): 517–26.

Sandler, R. and Smith, A.D. (1991) Coexistence of GABA and glutamate in mossy fiber terminals of the primate hippocampus: an ultrastructural study. J Comp Neurol 303(2):177–92.

Santhakumar, V. and Soltesz, I. (2004) Plasticity of interneuronal species diversity and parameter variance in neurological diseases. Trends Neurosci 27(8):504–10.

Santhakumar, V., Aradi, I. and Soltesz, I. (2005) Role of mossy fiber sprouting and mossy cell loss in hyperexcitability: a network model of the dentate gyrus incorporating cell types and axonal topography. J Neurophysiol 93(1):437–53.

Sayin, U., Osting, S., Hagen, J., Rutecki, P. and Sutula, T. (2003) Spontaneous seizures and loss of axo-axonic and axo-somatic inhibition induced by repeated brief seizures in kindled rats. J Neurosci 23(7): 2759–68.

Schneider, E.L., Kram, D., Nakanishi, Y., Monticone, R.E., Tice, R.R., Gilman, B.A. and Nieder, M.L. (1979) The effect of aging on sister chromatid exchange. Mech Ageing Dev 9(3–4):303–311.

Schwarzer, C. and Sperk, G. (1995) Hippocampal granule cells express glutamic acid decarboxylase-67 after limbic seizures in the rat. Neuroscience 69(3):705–9.

Shah, M.M., Anderson, A.E., Leung, V., Lin, X. and Johnston, D. (2004) Seizure-induced plasticity of h channels in entorhinal cortical layer III pyramidal neurons. Neuron 44(3):495–508.

Sharp, A.A., O'Neil, M.B., Abbott, L.F. and Marder, E. (1993) The dynamic clamp: artificial conductances in biological neurons. Trends Neurosci 16(10):389–94.

Sheng, H.Z., Lin, P.X. and Nelson, P.G. (1995) Combinatorial expression of immediate early genes in single neurons. Brain Res 30(2):196–202.

Shepherd, G.M. (1991) Foundations of the Neuron Doctrine. New York, Oxford: Oxford University Press.

Sherr, E.H. (2003) The ARX story (epilepsy, mental retardation, autism, and cerebral malformations): one gene leads to many phenotypes. Curr Opin Pediatr 15(6):567–71.

Shigemoto, R., Kulik, A., Roberts, J.D., Ohishi, H., Nusser, Z., Kaneko, T. and Somogyi, P. (1996) Target-cell-specific concentration of a metabotropic glutamate receptor in the presynaptic active zone. Nature 381(6582):523–5.

Shimamura, K., Hartigan, D.J., Martinez, S., Puelles, L. and Rubenstein, J.L. (1995) Longitudinal organization of the anterior neural plate and neural tube. Development 121(12):3923–33.

Sidman, R.L. and Rakic, P. (1973) Neuronal migration, with special reference to developing human brain: a review. Brain Res 62(1):1–35.

Sik, A., Ylinen, A., Penttonen, M. and Buzsáki, G. (1994) Inhibitory CA1-CA3-hilar region feedback in the hippocampus. Science 265(5179): 1722–4.

Sik, A., Penttonen, M., Ylinen, A. and Buzsáki, G. (1995) Hippocampal CA1 interneurons: an in vivo intracellular labeling study. J Neurosci 15(10):6651–65.

Sik, A., Penttonen, M. and Buzsáki, G. (1997) Interneurons in the hippocampal dentate gyrus: an in vivo intracellular study. Eur J Neurosci 9(3):573–88.

Simon, A., Olah, S., Molnar, G., Szabadics, J. and Tamas, G. (2005) Gap-junctional coupling between neurogliaform cells and various inter-neuron types in the neocortex. J Neurosci 25(27):6278–6285.

Simon, D.K., Lin, M.T., Zheng, L., Liu, G.J., Ahn, C.H., Kim, L.M., Mauck, W.M., Twu, F., Beal, M.F. and Johns, D.R. (2004) Somatic mitochondrial DNA mutations in cortex and substantia nigra in aging and Parkinson's disease. Neurobiol Aging 25(1):71–81.

Slater, P.J.B. and Halliday, T.R. (1994) Behavior and Evolution. Cambridge: Cambridge University Press.

Sloviter, R.S., Dichter, M.A., Rachinsky, T.L., Dean, E., Goodman, J.H., Sollas, A.L. and Martin, D.L. (1996) Basal expression and induction of glutamate decarboxylase and GABA in excitatory granule cells of the rat and monkey hippocampal dentate gyrus. J Comp Neurol 373(4):593–618.

Soltesz, I. and Deschênes, M. (1993) Low- and high-frequency membrane potential oscillations during theta activity in CA1 and CA3 pyramidal neurons of the rat hippocampus under ketamine-xylazine anesthesia. J Neurophysiol 97–116.

Soltesz, I. and Nusser, Z. (2001) Neurobiology. Background inhibition to the fore. Nature 409:24–7.

Somogyi, P. (1977) A specific "axo-axonal" interneuron in the visual cortex of the rat. Brain Res 136:345–50

Somogyi, P., Freund, T.F. and Cowey, A. (1982) The axo-axonic interneuron in the cerebral cortex of the rat, cat and monkey. Neuroscience 7(11):2577–607.

Somogyi, P., Kisvárday, Z.F., Martin, K.A. and Whitteridge D. (1983) Synaptic connections of morphologically identified and physiologically character-ized large basket cells in the striate cortex of cat. Neuroscience 10(2): 261–94.

Somogyi, P., Nunzi, M.G., Gorio, A. and Smith, A.D. (1983) A new type of specific interneuron in the monkey hippocampus forming synapses exclusively with the axon initial segments of pyramidal cells. Brain Res 259(1):137–42.

Somogyi, P., Hodgson, A.J., Smith, A.D., Nunzi, M.G., Gorio, A. and Wu, J.Y. (1984) Different populations of GABAergic neurons in the visual cortex and hippocampus of cat contain somatostatin- or cholecystokinin-immunoreactive material. J Neurosci 4(10):2590–603.

Somogyi, P. and Soltesz, I. (1986) Immunogold demonstration of GABA in synaptic terminals of intracellularly recorded, horseradish peroxidase-filled basket cells and clutch cells in the cat's visual cortex. Neuroscience 19(4):1051–65.

Somogyi, P., Fritschy, J.M., Benke, D., Roberts, J.D. and Sieghart, W. (1996) The gamma 2 subunit of the GABAA receptor is concentrated in synaptic junctions containing the alpha 1 and beta 2/3 subunits in hip-pocampus, cerebellum and globus pallidus. Neuropharmacology 35(9–10):1425–44.

Somogyi, P., Tamas, G., Lujan, R. and Buhl, E.H. (1998) Salient features of synaptic organisation in the cerebral cortex. Brain Res Rev 26(2–3): 113–35.

Somogyi, P., Dalezios, Y., Lujan, R., Roberts, J.D., Watanabe, M. and Shigemoto, R. (2003) High level of mGluR7 in the presynaptic active zones of select populations of GABAergic terminals innervating interneurons in the rat hippocampus. Eur J Neurosci 17(12):2503–20.

Somogyi, P. and Klausberger, T. (2005) Defined types of cortical interneurone structure space and spike timing in the hippocampus. J Physiol 562(Pt 1):9–26.

Soria, J.M. and Valdeolmillos, M. (2002) Receptor-activated calcium signals in tangentially migrating cortical cells. Cereb Cortex 12(8):831–9.

Soriano, E., Cobas, A. and Fairen, A. (1986) Asynchronism in the neuro-genesis of GABAergic and non-GABAergic neurons in the mouse hippocampus. Brain Res 395(1):88–92.

Soto-Trevino, C., Thoroughman, K.A., Marder, E. and Abbott, L.F. (2001) Activity-dependent modification of inhibitory synapses in models of rhythmic neural networks. Nat Neurosci 4(3):297–303.

Sporns, O. and Zwi, J.D. (2004) The small world of the cerebral cortex. Neuroinformatics 2(2):145–62.

Sprent, P. and Smeeton, N.C. (2001) Applied Non-Parametric Statistical Methods. London: Chapman & Hall.

Spruston, N., Lubke, J. and Frotscher, M. (1997) Interneurons in the stratum lucidum of the rat hippocampus: an anatomical and electrophysiological characterization. J Comp Neurol 385(3):427–40.

Stenman, J.M., Wang, B. and Campbell, K. (2003) Tlx controls proliferation and patterning of lateral telencephalic progenitor domains. J Neurosci 23(33):10568–76.

Stephan, K.E., Hilgetag, C.C., Burns, G.A., O'Neill, M.A., Young, M.P. and Kotter, R. (2000) Computational analysis of functional connectivity between areas of primate cerebral cortex. Philos Trans R Soc Lond B Biol Sci 355(1393):111–26.

Steriade, M., Amzica, F. and Contreras, D. (1996) Synchronization of fast (30–40 Hz) spontaneous cortical rhythms during brain activation. J Neurosci 16(1):392–417.

Steriade, M., Timofeev, I., Durmuller, N. and Grenier, F. (1998) Dynamic properties of corticothalamic neurons and local cortical interneurons generating fast rhythmic (30–40 Hz) spike bursts. J Neurophysiol 79(1):483–90.

Steriade, M. (2004) Neocortical cell classes are flexible entities. Nat Rev Neurosci 5(2):121–34.

Stevens, C.F. (1998) Neuronal diversity: too many cell types for comfort? Curr Biol 8(20):R708–10

Striedter, G.F. (2005) Principles of Brain Evolution. Sunderland, Mass.: Sinauer Associates.

Strogatz, S.H. (2001) Exploring complex networks. Nature 410:268–76.

Stuart, G.R., Oda, Y., de Boer, J.G. and Glickman BW. (2000) Mutation frequency and specificity with age in liver, bladder and brain of lacI transgenic mice. Genetics 154(3):1291–300.

Sur, M., Merzenich, M.M. and Kaas, J.H. (1980) Magnification, receptive-field area, and "hypercolumn" size in areas 3b and 1 of somatosensory cortex in owl monkeys. J Neurophysiol 44(2):295–311.

Sussel, L., Marin, O., Kimura, S. and Rubenstein, J.L. (1999) Loss of Nkx2.1 homeobox gene function results in a ventral to dorsal molecular respec-ification within the basal telencephalon: evidence for a transformation of the pallidum into the striatum. Development 126(15):3359–70.

Swiger, R.R., Cosentino, L., Shima, N., Bielas, J.H., Cruz-Munoz, W. and Heddle, J.A. (1999) The cII locus in the MutaMouse system. Environ Mol Mutagen 34(2–3):201–7.

Swiger, R.R., Cosentino, L., Masumura, K.I., Nohmi, T. and Heddle, J.A. (2001) Further characterization and validation of gpt delta transgenic mice for quantifying somatic mutations in vivo. Environ Mol Mutagen 37(4):297–303.

Szabadics, J., Lorincz, A. and Tamas, G. (2001) Beta and gamma frequency synchronization by dendritic gabaergic synapses and gap junctions in a network of cortical interneurons. J Neurosci 21(15):5824–31.

Szentágothai, J. and Arbib, M.A. (1974) Conceptual models of neural organization. Neurosci Res Program Bull 12(3):305–510.

Szentágothai J (1978) The Ferrier Lecture, 1977. The neuron network of the cerebral cortex: a functional interpretation. Proc R Soc Lond B Biol Sci 201(1144):219–48.

Szentágothai J (1983) The modular architectonic principle of neural centers. Rev Physiol Biochem Pharmacol 98:11–61.

Szentágothai J (1990) "Specificity versus (quasi-) randomness" revisited. Acta Morphol Hung 38(3–4):159–67.

Takahashi, J., Palmer, T.D. and Gage, F.H. (1999) Retinoic acid and neurotrophins collaborate to regulate neurogenesis in adult-derived neural stem cell cultures. J Neurobiol 38(1):65–81.

Tamas, G., Buhl, E.H., Lorincz, A. and Somogyi, P. (2000) Proximally targeted GABAergic synapses and gap junctions synchronize cortical interneurons. Nat Neurosci 3(4):366–71.

Tamas, G., Lorincz, A., Simon, A. and Szabadics, J. (2003) Identified sources and targets of slow inhibition in the neocortex. Science 299(5614): 1902–5.

Tecott, L.H., Maricq, A.V. and Julius, D. (1993) Nervous system distribution of the serotonin 5-HT3 receptor mRNA. Proc Natl Acad Sci U S A 90(4):1430–4.

Thomson, A.M., Bannister, A.P., Hughes, D.I. and Pawelzik, H. (2000) Differential sensitivity to Zolpidem of IPSPs activated by morphologically identified CA1 interneurons in slices of rat hippocampus. Eur J Neurosci 12(2):425–36.

Thomson, F.C. (1997) Names: The keys to biodiversity. In: Biodiversity II: Understanding and Protecting Our Biological Resources, eds. Reaka-Kudla, M.L., Wilson, D.E. and Wilson, E.O. pp. 199–213. Washington, DC: Joseph Henry Press.

Tierney, J. (1984) Paul Erdos is in town. His brain is open. Science 84:40–47.

Tiesinga, P.H. and Jose, J.V. (2000) Robust gamma oscillations in networks of inhibitory hippocampal interneurons. Network 11(1):1–23.

Toledo-Rodriguez, M., Blumenfeld, B., Wu, C., Luo, J., Attali, B., Goodman, P. and Markram, H. (2004) Correlation maps allow neuronal electrical properties to be predicted from single-cell gene expression profiles in rat neocortex. Cereb Cortex 14(12):1310–27.

Toth, K. and Freund, T.F. (1992) Calbindin D28k-containing nonpyramidal cells in the rat hippocampus: their immunoreactivity for GABA and projection to the medial septum. Neuroscience 49(4):793–805.

Toth, K., Borhegyi, Z. and Freund, T.F. (1993) Postsynaptic targets of GABAergic hippocampal neurons in the medial septum-diagonal band of broca complex. J Neurosci 13(9):3712–24.

Toth, Z., Hollrigel, G.S., Gorcs, T. and Soltesz, I. (1997a) Instantaneous perturbation of dentate interneuronal networks by a pressure wave-transient delivered to the neocortex. J Neurosci 17(21):8106–17.

Toth, K., Freund, T.F. and Miles, R. (1997b) Disinhibition of rat hippocampal pyramidal cells by GABAergic afferents from the septum. J Physiol 500(Pt 2):463–74.

Traub, R.D., Spruston, N., Soltesz, I., Konnerth, A., Whittington, M.A. and Jefferys, G.R. (1998) Gamma-frequency oscillations: a neuronal population phenomenon, regulated by synaptic and intrinsic cellular processes, and inducing synaptic plasticity. Prog Neurobiol 55(6):563–75.

Traub, R.D., Jeffereys, J.G.R. and Whittington, M.A. (1999) Fast Oscillations in Cortical Circuits. Cambridge, Mass.: MIT Press.

Traub, R.D., Contreras, D., Cunningham, M.O., Murray, H., Lebeau, F.E., Roopun, A., Bibbig, A., Wilent, W.B., Higley, M. and Whittington MA. (2005) A single-column thalamocortical network model exhibiting gamma oscillations, sleep spindles and epileptogenic bursts. J Neurophysiol 2004 Nov 3 [Epub ahead of print]

Turrigiano, G.G. and Nelson, S.B. (2000) Hebb and homeostasis in neuronal plasticity. Curr Opin Neurobiol. 10(3):358–364.

Turrigiano, G., Abbott, L.F. and Marder, E. (1994) Activity-dependent changes in the intrinsic properties of cultured neurons. Science 264(5161):974–7.

Turrigiano, G.G., Leslie, K.R., Desai, N.S., Rutherford, L.C. and Nelson, S.B. (1998) Activity-dependent scaling of quantal amplitude in neocortical neurons. Nature 391:892–6.

Turrigiano, G.G. and Nelson, S.B. (1998) Thinking globally, acting locally: AMPA receptor turnover and synaptic strength. Neuron 21(5):933–5.

Turrigiano, G.G. and Nelson, S.B. (2004) Homeostatic plasticity in the developing nervous system. Nat Rev Neurosci 5(2):97–107.

Valcanis, H. and Tan, S.S. (2003) Layer specification of transplanted interneurons in developing mouse neocortex. J Neurosci 23(12): 5113–22.

Valverde, F. (1971) Short axon neuronal subsystems in the visual cortex of the monkey. Int J Neurosci 1: 181–197.

Van der Loos, H. and Woolsey, T.A. (1973) Somatosensory cortex: structural alterations following early injury to sense organs. Science 179(71):395–8.

van Groen, T. and Wyss, J.M. (1990) Extrinsic projections from area CA1 of the rat hippocampus: olfactory, cortical, subcortical, and bilateral hippocampal formation projections. J Comp Neurol 302(3):515–28.

Vanderwolf, C.H. (1969) Hippocampal electrical activity and voluntary movement in the rat. Electroencephalogr Clin Neurophysiol 26(4): 407–18.

Veldic, M., Caruncho, H.J., Liu, W.S., Davis, J., Satta, R., Grayson, D.R., Guidotti, A. and Costa, E. (2004) DNA-methyltransferase 1 mRNA is selectively overexpressed in telencephalic GABAergic interneurons of schizophrenia brains. Proc Natl Acad Sci U S A 101(1):348–53.

Venance, L., Rozov, A., Blatow, M., Burnashev, N., Feldmeyer, D. and Monyer, H. (2000) Connexin expression in electrically coupled postnatal rat brain neurons. Proc Natl Acad Sci U S A 97(18):10260–5.

Vergara, C., Latorre, R., Marrion, N.V. and Adelman, J.P. (1998) Calcium-activated potassium channels. Curr Opin Neurobiol 8(3):321–9.

Vida, I., Halasy, K., Szinyei, C., Somogyi, P. and Buhl EH. (1998) Unitary IPSPs evoked by interneurons at the stratum radiatum-stratum lacunosum-moleculare border in the CA1 area of the rat hippocampus in vitro. J Physiol 506 (Pt 3):755–73.

Walker, M.C., Ruiz, A. and Kullmann, D.M. (2001) Monosynaptic GABAergic signaling from dentate to CA3 with a pharmacological and physiological profile typical of mossy fiber synapses. Neuron 29(3):703–15.

Wang, X.J. and Buzsáki, G. (1996) Gamma oscillation by synaptic inhibition in a hippocampal interneuronal network model. J Neurosci 16(20): 6402–13.

Wang, X.J., Tegner, J., Constantinidis, C. and Goldman-Rakic, P.S. (2004) Division of labor among distinct subtypes of inhibitory neurons in a cortical microcircuit of working memory. Proc Natl Acad Sci U S A 101(5):1368–73.

Wassle, H., Peichl, L. and Boycott, B.B. (1981) Dendritic territories of cat retinal ganglion cells. Nature 292(5821):344–5.

Watt, A.J., van Rossum, M.C., MacLeod, K.M., Nelson, S.B. and Turrigiano, G.G. (2000) Activity coregulates quantal AMPA and NMDA currents at neocortical synapses. Neuron 26(3):659–70.

Watts, D.J. and Strogatz, S.H. (1998) Collective dynamics of 'small-world' networks. Nature 393(6684):440–2.

Watts, D.J. (1999) Small Worlds: The dynamics of networks between order and randomness. Princeton, N.J.: Princeton University Press.

Weiner, J. (1994) The Beak of the Finch. New York: Vintage Books, Random House.

Weiss, K.M. (2005) The phenogenetic logic of life. Nat Rev Genet 6(1):36–45.

White, J.A., Chow, C.C., Ritt, J., Soto-Trevino, C. and Kopell, N. (1998) Synchronization and oscillatory dynamics in heterogeneous, mutually inhibited neurons. J Comput Neurosci 5(1):5–16.

Whittington, M.A., Traub, R.D., Kopell, N., Ermentrout, B. and Buhl, E.H. (2000) Inhibition-based rhythms: experimental and mathematical observations on network dynamics. Int J Psychophysiol 38(3):315–36.

Whittington, M.A. and Traub, R.D. (2003) Interneuron diversity series: inhibitory interneurons and network oscillations in vitro. Trends Neurosci 26(12):676–82.

Wichterle, H., Alvarez-Dolado, M., Erskine, L. and Alvarez-Buylla, A. (2003) Permissive corridor and diffusible gradients direct medial ganglionic eminence cell migration to the neocortex. Proc Natl Acad Sci USA 100(2):727–732.

Wichterle, H., Turnbull, D.H., Nery, S., Fishell, G. and Alvarez-Buylla, A. (2001) In utero fate mapping reveals distinct migratory pathways and fates of neurons born in the mammalian basal forebrain. Development 128(19):3759–71.

Wiesel, T.N. and Gilbert, C.D. (1983) The Sharpey-Schafer lecture. Morphological basis of visual cortical function. Q J Exp Physiol 68(4):525–43.

Wilson, E.O. and Bossert, W.H. (1971) A Primer of Population Biology. Sunderland, Mass.: Sinauer Associates.

Wilson, E.O. (1992) The Diversity of Life. New York: W.W. Norton & Co.

Wilson, M.A. and McNaughton, B.L. (1993) Dynamics of the hippocampal ensemble code for space. Science 261(5124):1055–8.

Wilson, R.I., Kunos, G. and Nicoll, R.A. (2001) Presynaptic specificity of endocannabinoid signaling in the hippocampus. Neuron 31(3):453–62.

Wisden, W., Laurie, D.J., Monyer, H. and Seeburg, P.H. (1992) The distribution of 13 GABAA receptor subunit mRNAs in the rat brain. I. Telencephalon, diencephalon, mesencephalon. J Neurosci 12(3): 1040–62.

Wittner, L., Magloczky, Z., Borhegyi, Z., Halasz, P., Toth, S., Eross, L., Szabo, Z. and Freund, T.F. (2001) Preservation of perisomatic inhibitory input of granule cells in the epileptic human dentate gyrus. Neuroscience 108(4):587–600.

Wittner, L., Eross, L., Szabo, Z., Toth, S., Czirjak, S., Halasz, P. and Freund, T.F. and Magloczky, Z.S. (2002) Synaptic reorganization of calbindin-positive neurons in the human hippocampal CA1 region in temporal lobe epilepsy. Neuroscience 115(3):961–78.

Wonders, C. and Anderson, S. (2005) Beyond migration: Dlxl regulates interneuron differentiation. Nat Neurosci 8(8):979–981.

Wuchty, S. (2001) Scale-free behavior in protein domain networks. Mol Biol Evol 18(9):1694–702.

Xu, Q., Cobos, I., De La Cruz, E., Rubenstein, J.L. and Anderson, S.A. (2004) Origins of cortical interneuron subtypes. J Neurosci 24(11): 2612–22.

Ylinen, A., Soltesz, I., Bragin, A., Penttonen, M., Sik, A. and Buzsáki, G. (1995) Intracellular correlates of hippocampal theta rhythm in identified pyramidal cells, granule cells, and basket cells. Hippocampus 5(1):78–90.

Yoshimura, S., Takagi, Y., Harada, J., Teramoto, T., Thomas, S.S., Waeber, C., Bakowska, J.C., Breakefield, X.O. and Moskowitz, M.A. (2001) FGF-2 regulation of neurogenesis in adult hippocampus after brain injury. Proc Natl Acad Sci U S A 98(10):5874–9.

Zappone, C.A. and Sloviter, R.S. (2001) Commissurally projecting inhibitory interneurons of the rat hippocampal dentate gyrus: a colocalization study of neuronal markers and the retrograde tracer Fluoro-gold. J Comp Neurol 441(4):324–44.

Zar, J. (1999) Biostatistical Analysis. Englewood Cliffs, N.J.: Prentice-Hall.

Zawar, C., Plant, T.D., Schirra, C., Konnerth, A. and Neumcke, B. (1999) Cell-type specific expression of ATP-sensitive potassium channels in the rat hippocampus. J Physiol 514 (Pt 2):327–41.

Zhang, X.B., Urlando, C., Tao, K.S. and Heddle, J.A. (1995) Factors affecting somatic mutation frequencies in vivo. Mutat Res 338(1–6): 189–201.

Zhao, Y., Marin, O., Hermesz, E., Powell, A., Flames, N., Palkovits, M., Rubenstein, J.L. and Westphal, H. (2003) The LIM-homeobox gene Lhx8 is required for the development of many cholinergic neurons in the mouse forebrain. Proc Natl Acad Sci U S A 100(15):9005–10.

Zhu, Y., Li, H., Zhou, L., Wu, J.Y. and Rao, Y. (1999) Cellular and molecular guidance of GABAergic neuronal migration from an extracortical origin to the neocortex. Neuron 23(3):473–85.

Index